# Praise for *Tai Chi for Balance*

"Falls are devastating not only for older adults, but for middle-aged and younger people with musculoskeletal conditions such as arthritis. Even the fear of potentially falling can adversely impact mental health and profoundly reduce quality of life. Chris Cinnamon has created an evidence-based program to help improve balance and stability while restoring peoples' confidence and trust in their own bodies. *Tai Chi for Balance* is well researched and easy to read with clear explanations of both the exercises and the underlying science. This book will be an outstanding resource for anyone concerned about falling."

Kharma Foucher, MD, PhD, Associate Professor, Dept. of Kinesiology and Nutrition, University of Illinois at Chicago

\* \* \*

"Chris Cinnamon's *Tai Chi for Balance* is a much-needed guide for anyone who has ever struggled with gait unsteadiness and falls. It provides a systematic approach on how Tai Chi can be incorporated into a regular routine to improve balance and prevent falls. The explanations on how and why Tai Chi works are based on the medical literature and the author's extensive experience in teaching adults. With its straightforward style and helpful illustrations, the book is easy to follow and fun to read. This is a wonderful resource for my patients!"

Jinny Tavee, MD, Chief of Neurology, National Jewish Health

\* \* \*

"Next time I'm asked for recommendations on how to stay healthy past 60, I'll tell them to read Chris Cinnamon's *Tai Chi for Balance*. Falling is a major medical issue for older adults, resulting in serious injuries and loss of independence. *Tai Chi for Balance* provides a solution. Chris guides you through an easy-to-follow Tai Chi exercise program, based on sound science, with a clear emphasis on how to increase stability and avoid falls. A must read for all adults over 60."

Christine Rosenbloom, PhD, author, *Food and Fitness after 50*

\* \* \*

"*Tai Chi for Balance: How to Stay on Your Feet and Avoid Falls* is a valuable book for older adults seeking the benefits of Tai Chi for falls prevention. Chris Cinnamon provides a useful summary of the scientific evidence and key concepts before guiding the reader through Tai Chi for Balance exercises. This book will help older adults prevent falls and gain all the other benefits of Tai Chi for their health and wellbeing."

Dr. Samuel Nyman, Head, Department of Psychology, University of Winchester

\* \* \*

"Improve your balance and stability. You can do it! In *Tai Chi for Balance*, Chris Cinnamon presents a detailed, step by step movement program to do just that. It's easy to follow and includes excellent resources to enhance your experience. Having personally regained my balance and ability to walk through Tai Chi, I know that Chris' approach is sound and effective. Say yes to better balance. *Tai Chi for Balance* will be your guide."

Arlene Faulk, M.A., Faulk Tai Chi owner and head instructor, author, *Walking on Pins and Needles: A Memoir of Chronic Resilience in the Face of Multiple Sclerosis*

\* \* \*

"*Tai Chi for Balance* provides a fantastic new resource for older adults and those who work with them. Infused with detailed explanations founded on science and experience, Chris teaches readers the importance of low-impact exercise and deliberate cultivation of body awareness for avoiding falls. Read *Tai Chi for Balance* and you'll find ease of understanding and application firmly supported at its foundation with why Tai Chi matters in the lives of individuals and healthcare at large."

Karrie L. Hamstra-Wright, PhD, Clinical Professor, Department of Kinesiology and Nutrition, University of Illinois at Chicago

\* \* \*

"In *Tai Chi for Balance*, Chris Cinnamon does a masterful job showing how Tai Chi can benefit anyone on the path of healthy aging. And avoiding falls is a key! Chris book shows you how."

"As a teacher, what I love most about this book is that it's not just for students; it's a terrific resource for Tai Chi and Qigong instructors who want to give additional support to their students."

"Qigong and Tai Chi saved me from major depression and chronic pain, so that's what I've focused my teaching on. Even though I have thousands of online students all over the world, I'm not an expert in using Tai Chi for balance. That's where Chris' book comes in. I'm grateful that he has put so much time and energy into sharing his expertise. He has made it easier for me to serve my own students."

"I wholeheartedly recommend *Tai Chi for Balance* to anyone seeking to safeguard their golden years, as well as those who are helping them along that path. If you teach Tai Chi or Qigong, then this book should be on your shelf, and your students' shelves."

Anthony Korahais, author, *Flowing Zen: Finding True Healing with Qigong*

# Tai Chi for Balance

# Tai Chi for Balance

## How to Stay on Your Feet and Avoid Falls

Chris Cinnamon, JD, MS, CEP

Illustrated by Elizabeth Moss, MS

Copyright © 2023 Christopher C. Cinnamon

All rights reserved. No part of this publication and the accompanying videos may be reproduced, distributed, or transmitted in any form or by any means, including photocopying, recording, or other electronic or mechanical methods, without the prior written permission of the publisher, except in the case of brief quotations embodied in critical reviews and other noncommercial uses permitted by copyright law. For permission requests, write to the publisher, addressed "Attention: Permission Coordinator," at the following address.

CTC Publishing
180 West Washington Ave.
Suite 900
Chicago, Illinois 60602
info@chicagotaichi.org

www.chicagotaichi.org

First Edition

ISBN 978-1-7343369-3-1

Before engaging in any new exercise program, including Tai Chi for Balance, you should consult with an appropriate medical professional and receive clearance to engage in exercise. Any exercise presents a risk of injury. To minimize injury risk in Tai Chi for Balance, you should: (i) obtain clearance from your medical professional; (ii) follow all instructions in this book; (iii) stop any exercise that causes discomfort or pain; and (iv) consult with an appropriate medical professional if the pain persists.

This book is written as a source of information only and is not intended as a substitute for medical advice.

Although the author and publisher have made reasonable efforts to ensure that the information in this book was correct when published, the author and publisher expressly disclaim any liability to any party for any loss, damage, or disruption caused by any errors or omissions.

# Contents

Acknowledgments ........................................................................................... vii
Introduction .................................................................................................... 1
   Why I Wrote This Book ............................................................................. 1
   Who Can Benefit from This Book ............................................................. 3
   Overview: The Tai Chi for Balance System ............................................... 4
   How to Use This Book ............................................................................... 6
   The Tai Chi for Balance Learning Approach ............................................. 8
Part 1 The Foundation: Before We Start Moving ........................................ 11
   Chapter 1 Aging and Falling: Bad News and Good News ...................... 13
      The Bad News: Older Adults and Falling ............................................ 14
      The Good News: Falls are Preventable ................................................ 18
      The Science: Tai Chi and Falls Prevention .......................................... 19
      Chapter Wrap-Up ................................................................................. 24
   Chapter 2 Key Concepts ........................................................................... 33
      Stability ................................................................................................ 33
      Center of Gravity ................................................................................. 35
      Base of Support ................................................................................... 37
      How to Increase Stability .................................................................... 39
      Whole Body Awareness ...................................................................... 45
      Precise Posture Control ....................................................................... 46
      Chapter Wrap-Up ................................................................................. 47
   Chapter 3 The Two Rules ......................................................................... 49
      Rule #1: The 70% Rule ....................................................................... 49
      Rule #2: The Don't Cause Pain Rule ................................................... 51
      Chapter Wrap-Up ................................................................................. 53
   Chapter 4 Neutral Posture, Feeling Your Feet, and Feeling Your Center ........ 55
      Neutral Posture .................................................................................... 55
      Feeling Your Feet ................................................................................ 62
      Exercise 1: Feeling Your Feet ............................................................. 63

  Feeling Your Center .................................................................................... 68

  Exercise 2: Feeling Your Center .................................................................. 69

  Exercise 3: Feeling Your Feet and Center ...................................................74

  Chapter Wrap-up ........................................................................................ 80

**Part 2 Beginning to Move: Vertical Circles** ................................................... 83

 Chapter 5 Connecting the Bottom to the Top: The Kwa Squat .............................. 85

  Exercise 4: Finding Your *Kwa* .................................................................... 86

  Basic Elements ............................................................................................87

  Tips and Common Errors ........................................................................... 88

  Exercise 5: The Kwa Squat.......................................................................... 90

  Exercise 6: Kwa Squat + Feeling Your Feet and Center ...............................91

  Chapter Wrap-Up........................................................................................93

 Chapter 6 Adding the Arms: Vertical Circles ......................................................95

  Basic Elements ............................................................................................95

  Tips and Common Errors ........................................................................... 98

  Exercise 7: Vertical Circles........................................................................ 100

  Exercise 8: Vertical Circles + Feeling Your Feet and Center ......................102

  Chapter Wrap-up ...................................................................................... 104

 Chapter 7 Circle #1: Vertical Circles + Kwa Squat.............................................. 105

  Basic Elements .......................................................................................... 105

  Tips and Common Errors ..........................................................................109

  Exercise 9: Vertical Circles + Kwa Squat .................................................... 111

  Exercise 10: Vertical Circles + Kwa Squat + Feeling Your Feet and Center .... 113

  Chapter Wrap-up ...................................................................................... 115

 Chapter 8 Adding More Legs: The Weight Shift..................................................117

  The Tai Chi for Balance Stance.................................................................. 118

  Exercise 11: The Weight Shift ................................................................... 122

  Common Error .......................................................................................... 124

  Exercise 12: Weight Shift + Feeling Your Center ....................................... 125

  Exercise 13: Weight Shift + Feeling Your Feet and Center........................128

- Chapter Wrap-up .................................................................................. 130
- Chapter 9 Circle #2: Vertical Circles + Weight Shift ............................. 131
  - Basic Elements ................................................................................ 132
  - Tips and Common Errors ............................................................... 140
  - Exercise 14: Vertical Circles + Weight Shift .................................. 142
  - Exercise 15: Vertical Circles + Weight Shift + Feeling Your Feet and Center . 146
  - Chapter Wrap-up ............................................................................ 148
- Chapter 10 Adding Rotation: The Hip Turn .......................................... 149
  - The Two Fundamental Knee Alignments ....................................... 150
  - Adding Rotation: The Hip Turn + Kwa Fold .................................. 151
  - Basic Elements ................................................................................ 151
  - Tips and Common Errors ............................................................... 156
  - Exercise 16: Hip Turn + Kwa Fold .................................................. 158
  - Exercise 17: Weight Shift + Hip Turn ............................................. 161
  - Chapter Wrap-up ............................................................................ 164
- Chapter 11 Adding Rotation: Keeping the 4 Points Aligned ................. 165
  - Your 4 Points and How to Keep Them Aligned ............................. 165
  - Exercise 18: Weight Shift + Hip Turn + Keeping the 4 Points Aligned .......... 169
  - Exercise 19: Weight Shift + Hip Turn + Feeling Your Feet and Center .......... 172
  - Chapter Wrap-up ............................................................................ 174
- Chapter 12 Circle #3: Vertical Circles + Weight Shift + Hip Turn ......... 175
  - Basic Elements ................................................................................ 176
  - Learning Circle #3: The Four Checkpoints .................................... 184
  - Exercise 20: Vertical Circles + Weight Shift + Hip Turn ................ 189
  - Exercise 21: Vertical Circles + Weight Shift + Hip Turn + Feeling Your Feet and Center ................................................................................................. 192
  - Chapter Wrap-up ............................................................................ 194
- Chapter 13 Building Our Tai Chi for Balance Exercise Set: Circles #1 through #3 ............................................................................................................ 195
  - Exercise 22: Circles #1 through #3 .................................................. 197

**Part 3 Continuing to Move: Horizontal Circles** .................................................................. 205

    **Chapter 14 Circle #4: Horizontal Circles + Kwa Squat** .............................. 207

        Basic Elements ................................................................................................ 209

        Tips and Common Errors .............................................................................. 214

        Exercise 23: Horizontal Circles + Kwa Squat ............................................. 216

        Exercise 24: Horizontal Circles + Kwa Squat + Feeling Your Feet and Center ................................................................................................................. 218

        Chapter Wrap-up ............................................................................................ 220

    **Chapter 15 Circle #5: Horizontal Circles + Weight Shift + Hip Turn** ......... 221

        Basic Elements ................................................................................................ 221

        Tips and Common Errors .............................................................................. 229

        Exercise 25: Horizontal Circles + Weight Shift + Hip Turn ..................... 230

        Exercise 26: Horizontal Circles + Weight Shift + Hip Turn + Feeling Your Feet and Center ........................................................................................ 234

        Chapter Wrap-up ............................................................................................ 236

    **Chapter 16 Adding to Our Tai Chi for Balance Exercise Set: Circles #1 through #5** ..................................................................................................................... 237

        Exercise 27: Circles #1 through #5 .............................................................. 238

**Part 4 Completing the Set: Coronal Circles** ............................................................ 249

    **Chapter 17 Circle #6: Coronal Circles + Kwa Squat** ................................... 251

        Basic Elements ................................................................................................ 251

        Tips and Common Errors .............................................................................. 256

        Exercise 28: Coronal Circles + Kwa Squat ................................................. 258

        Exercise 29: Coronal Circles + Kwa Squat + Feeling Your Feet and Center ... 260

        Chapter Wrap-up ............................................................................................ 262

    **Chapter 18 Circle #7: Coronal Circles + Weight Shift + Hip Turn** ............ 263

        Basic Elements ................................................................................................ 264

        Tips and Common Errors .............................................................................. 272

        Exercise 30: Coronal Circles + Weight Shift + Hip Turn ......................... 273

        Exercise 31: Coronal Circles + Weight Shift + Hip Turn + Feeling Your Feet and Center ................................................................................................... 277

    Chapter Wrap-up .................................................................................... 279

    Chapter 19 Putting It All Together: Circles #1 through #7 ................................... 281

        Circles #1 through #7: Applying Key Principles ................................. 281

        Exercise 32: Circles #1 through #7 ........................................................ 283

Part 5 Stepping Up the Challenge: Tai Chi Walking ................................................ 297

    Chapter 20 Tai Chi Walking .................................................................................... 299

        Tai Chi Walking #1: Single Step Forward ........................................... 302

        Basic Elements ......................................................................................... 303

        Tips and Common Errors ..................................................................... 305

        Exercise 33: Tai Chi Walking; Single Step Forward ......................... 306

        Tai Chi Walking #2: Single Step Forward, Single Step Back, Single Step Forward .................................................................................................. 309

        Basic Elements: Single Step Forward, Single Step Back, Single Step Forward .................................................................................................. 309

        Tip ............................................................................................................... 314

        Exercise 34: Tai Chi Walking, Single Step Forward, Single Step Back, Single Step Forward ........................................................................................ 315

        Tai Chi Walking Exercise #3: Three Steps Forward and Sink ......... 318

        Basic Elements ......................................................................................... 320

        Tips and Common Errors ..................................................................... 323

        Exercise 35: Tai Chi Walking: Three Steps Forward and Sink ....... 324

        Chapter Wrap-up .................................................................................... 327

    Chapter 21 Conclusion: Next Steps in Staying on Your Feet and Avoiding Falls . 329

About the Author ................................................................................................... 333
About the Illustrator ............................................................................................... 334

# Acknowledgments

I extend my gratitude to many. First, to Master Bruce Frantzis, whose teaching led me to understand the potential of Tai Chi, Qigong, and meditation to support deep healing, vibrant health, spiritual growth, and— most importantly for this book—balance and stability, at all levels of our being. For more on Master Frantzis—including his books, online programs, and live trainings—go to [https://www.energyarts.com/](https://www.energyarts.com/).

To Kharma Foucher, MD, PhD, an expert in osteoarthritis and hip replacements and my academic advisor at University of Illinois at Chicago (UIC) from 2015–2017. Dr. Foucher leads UIC's Biomechanics and Clinical Outcomes Lab, where I worked as a graduate research assistant.

To my awesome illustrator, Elizabeth Moss.

To Annelise Senkowski, for ongoing support for this book, including serving as the female model for illustrations.

To my fantastic editor, Sarah Cisco, and my talented cover designer, Jess Estrella.

To my students and clients, who've engaged enthusiastically in the Tai Chi for Balance System and provided important feedback for refining the program.

# Introduction

## Why I Wrote This Book

I wrote this book to help you and other older adults stay on your feet and avoid falls.

Why? For several reasons.

**Falls are the #1 cause of injury in older adults.**

For older adults, injuries from falling include broken hips, shattered wrists, fractured ankles, broken and bruised ribs, cracked skulls, and traumatic brain injuries. Injuries like these cause pain and suffering, require costly medical treatment, and can require lengthy rehab to recover.

That's *if* you recover.

**Falls cause disability and loss of independence.**

Every year, thousands of older adults fall and *don't* recover. Falls often start a downward spiral leading to declining function, disability, and admission into assisted living facilities.

**Falls kill.**

Sadly, some falls are fatal. Falling is the #1 cause of death from injury in older adults. More than car wrecks or any other type of accident.

**Falls don't have to happen.** After all that bad news, there's good news. All leading medical authorities agree: *Falls are preventable.*

That's where I come in.

As an exercise physiologist and Head Instructor at the leading Tai Chi school in Chicago, my mission is to help adults achieve vibrant health. My students and clients include many older adults. **For older adults to enjoy vibrant health, they must avoid falling and the debilitating injuries that result.**

To address this risk, I developed and lead the **Tai Chi for Balance Program** at Chicago Tai Chi. Through my classes, workshops, and online courses, I've taught Tai Chi for Balance to thousands of older adults. It works. People get the training. They practice the exercises. And soon, they report feeling stable, secure, and confident on their feet.

And, most importantly, they avoid falls. Paul Brayman's story provides a powerful example.

**Paul Brayman's story.** Paul, a retired lawyer, attended one of my first Tai Chi for Balance Courses. The previous year, Paul fell, breaking an ankle.

During his first class, I observed Paul's stooped posture and tentative gait. Over the course of his training, Paul's posture gradually became more upright, and he walked with increasing confidence. What a transformation!

After completing the course, Paul tripped on the base of a construction sign near his home. Rather than falling hard on the concrete, he recovered, staying on his feet. He said, "Your Tai Chi for Balance exercises helped me be more aware of my feet and my posture and avoid falling."

That's Tai Chi for Balance in action!

By avoiding falls, like Paul did, my students and clients remain independent. They maintain, and even *gain* physical function, staying on the path to vibrant health.

Do you want that too?

*Introduction*

Of course! Who doesn't, right?

In this book, I show you how.

## Who Can Benefit from This Book

This book is for every adult at risk of injury from falling. That risk begins to increase around age 60. At age 65 and beyond, falling becomes the #1 cause of injury.

As an older adult, by following my Tai Chi for Balance System, you'll soon develop:

- **Whole Body Awareness**
- **Precise Posture Control**
- **Strong legs and hips**

Along the way, you'll pick up clear concepts and practical strategies for increasing stability and avoiding falls. These key program elements combine to help you feel stable, secure, and confident on your feet.

This book also serves as a resource for those working with older adults, including:

- Medical professionals
- Personal trainers
- Group exercise instructors
- Tai Chi instructors
- Caregivers
- Adult children of older adults

In this book, you'll find concepts, strategies, tools, and a complete Tai Chi-based exercise system to help patients, students, clients, and loved ones avoid falls.

I'm committed to helping you, and as many older adults as I can, enjoy an active, independent life—without the life-altering trauma and injuries of falling.

That's why I wrote this book.

# Overview: The Tai Chi for Balance System

The Tai Chi for Balance System distills key Tai Chi principles and movements into a low-impact, easy-to-follow, step-by-step program. The program also incorporates essential information about falls risks, key concepts from biomechanics, and practical falls-avoidance strategies. I've taught this material in live workshops, classes and private sessions, and to a growing US and international audience through my Online Tai Chi for Balance Course., available at https://www.chicagotaichi.org/tai-chi-for-balance-online-course/

In short, my Tai Chi for Balance System works. People get the training; they practice the material; and soon they feel stable, secure, and confident on their feet—avoiding falls and the life-altering consequences of falling.

Follow my guidance, and you'll experience that too.

**The Three Main Learning Objectives of Tai Chi for Balance**

I'll start with the big picture: the three main learning objectives of Tai Chi for Balance.

**Objective 1: Developing Whole Body Awareness.**

Throughout the Tai Chi for Balance program, I'll encourage you to feel your body. I call this ability to feel the body "Whole Body Awareness."

Why focus on developing Whole Body Awareness? Two big reasons.

First, most people don't consistently feel their bodies. Their minds are in their heads, with their awareness consumed with thoughts generated by parts of the brain. For most of us, it takes training and practice to get our minds out of our heads and become increasingly aware of what's going on in and around our bodies.

Second, Whole Body Awareness helps you avoid falls. When you become consistently aware of what's going on in and around your body, you gather lots of information that helps you stay on your feet.

*Introduction*

In Tai Chi for Balance, you'll discover how to become aware of your body with increasing consistency and clarity. As your Whole Body Awareness grows, you'll become more sensitive to internal and external sensations that signal an increased risk of falling.

**Objective 2: Developing Precise Posture Control**

With greater Whole Body Awareness, you'll increasingly feel your posture. By "posture," I mean how you align your body from your feet to the top of your head. With awareness of your posture, you'll develop skill at controlling your posture with increasing precision. The ultimate aim of Precise Posture Control is maintaining a posture that increases stability. **Maintaining a more stable structure makes you more resistant to falling.**

In Tai Chi for Balance, I guide you through specific techniques for feeling and adjusting your posture to maximize stability.

**Objective 3: Developing Strong Legs and Hips**

As you'll learn in Chapter 2, a leading risk factor for falls is loss of lower body strength as we age. The right kind of exercise reverses that, making your legs and hips stronger. The low-impact exercises in this book will do that for you, in a way that is comfortable and gradual, without the risk of strains or injuries associated with higher-impact exercise.

In this program, you'll learn a simplified, easy-to-follow, Tai Chi-based exercise set called Tai Chi Circling Hands®. Then we'll add a set of Tai Chi Walking exercises. With regular practice, this exercise system will strengthen your legs and hips as you become increasingly aware of your body and posture.

These three objectives—Whole Body Awareness, Precise Posture Control, and stronger legs and hips—combine to help you become stable, secure, and confident on your feet. Along the way, you'll learn practical strategies for avoiding falls.

**Tai Chi for Balance: Anyone Can Do It**

Tai Chi for Balance is a step-by-step system anyone can learn. You don't need a background in Tai Chi. You don't need to be physically fit. You don't need to have an ideal bodyweight. You don't need to think of yourself as "coordinated" or "graceful" or any other adjective used to describe how we move.

To succeed with Tai Chi for Balance, you need to make a commitment. Not a huge commitment, but a commitment, nonetheless. You need to commit to investing the time to learn and practice the Tai Chi for Balance System.

I know how overscheduled contemporary lives can be. Time is precious and increasingly scarce. When I say you need to invest time, I mean a little, not a lot. Once you learn the basics of this program, I recommend practicing 15–20 minutes per day, 4–5 days per week.

That small investment, just 15–20 minutes per day, 4–5 days per week, will reward you with **a wonderful sense of stability, security, and confidence on your feet**. You'll feel the satisfaction of taking a proactive approach to avoiding the life-altering consequences of a fall. You'll continue to experience the pleasure of an independent, active lifestyle.

You've already taken an important first step. You started this book. Good for you!

Here's how to use it.

## How to Use This Book

Through my workshops, classes, and my Online Tai Chi for Balance Course, I've honed a systematic approach to presenting this material. I follow that approach in this book.

I've organized this book into 5 parts, with a total of 21 chapters. The material builds sequentially, guiding you step-by-step through the principles and movements of the Tai Chi for Balance System.

**Part 1: The Foundation.** Chapters 1–4 establish the foundation for Tai Chi for Balance, introducing concepts, vocabulary, and material we use throughout the program. Chapter 1 presents an **overview of falls risks as we age** and the promising science supporting falls prevention. Chapter 2 covers key concepts from

*Introduction*

biomechanics, like **stability**, **center of gravity**, and **base of support**. Chapter 3 includes the "Two Rules" governing Tai Chi for Balance: the **70% Rule** and the **Don't Cause Pain Rule**. Chapter 4 introduces a way to stand called **Neutral Posture**, and how to feel your feet and your center.

**Part 2: Beginning to Move.** In Chapters 5–13, we begin to move, introducing most of the components of the Tai Chi for Balance Exercise Set. We'll cover movement components including the **Kwa Squat**, the **Kwa Fold**, the **Weight Shift**, the **Weight Shift + Hip Turn**, and **Vertical Circles**. We will put those movement components together into the first 3 movements of our 7-movement exercise set.

**Part 3: Continuing to Move**. Chapters 14–16 build upon Part 2, introducing another movement component, the **Horizontal Circle**. We then incorporate the Horizontal Circle into the 4th and 5th movements of our exercise set.

**Part 4: Completing the Set.** Chapters 17–19 add the final movement component, the **Coronal Circle**, incorporating that into the 6th and 7th movements of our exercise set.

By Chapter 19, we will be ready to put it all together, performing a complete set of Tai Chi Circling Hands. A full set involves performing each of the 7 movements 20 times, for a total of 140 movements. That's about 15 minutes of low-impact, whole body exercise, all focused on helping you develop:

- Whole Body Awareness
- Precise Posture Control
- Strong legs and hips

In doing so, you become more stable and secure on your feet and resistant to falls.

**Part 5: Stepping up the Challenge.** I conclude the program in Chapters 20 – 21. Chapter 20 introduces the final component of the Tai Chi for Balance System: Tai Chi Walking. The three exercises in this chapter build upon all the previous material, training you to become more stable and resistant to falls. Chapter 21 concludes with my recommendations on what to do after you finish this book.

# The Tai Chi for Balance Learning Approach

In this book, I guide you through Tai Chi for Balance with a systematic, step-by-step learning approach.

First, we learn movement components and related principles and techniques. Then we combine those movement components into whole-body movements. Then we connect those movements into a sequence of movements. Over Parts 2–4, we build our movement sequence into the 7-movement exercise set called Tai Chi Circling Hands.

I introduce each new movement with a **Basic Elements** section, breaking down the movement into its component parts. Most movements include a section on **Tips and Common Errors** to help guide your learning. I then lead you through a series of progressive **Exercises**, helping you to develop skill in performing the movements while monitoring an increasing number of "moving parts."

Each **Exercise** concludes with a **Practice Recommendation** to follow before proceeding.

**Online Practice Videos**

To help support your practice, you have access to a library of **online practice videos**. Just press play and follow me!

You can find links to those videos at the beginning of the applicable exercises.

**Online Tai Chi for Balance Course and Live Training**

As an additional resource, many of my workshop attendees, students, and clients join my Online Tai Chi for Balance Course. This comprehensive video course, with students enrolled across the US and internationally, provides video lessons and guided practices covering all the material presented in this book. The video course offers an effective additional resource to support home study. For more information and to purchase immediate access to the course, go to https://www.chicagotaichi.org/tai-chi-for-balance-online-course/

*Introduction*

I periodically offer live Tai Chi for Balance courses and workshops you can attend online or in-person. To receive updates about these opportunities and other opportunities to train with me, go to www.chicagotaichi.org and join our email list.

---

**Practice Note: Master Bruce Frantzis and Tai Chi Circling Hands**

In Tai Chi for Balance, you will learn a movement set called Tai Chi Circling Hands ("Circling Hands" for short). My main teacher, Master Bruce Frantzis, developed Tai Chi Circling Hands, incorporating key Tai Chi movement components into an easy-to-learn exercise system. Master Frantzis has generously granted his permission for me to use Tai Chi Circling Hands in this book.

I chose Circling Hands as the basis for the Tai Chi for Balance System for three main reasons: (1) It incorporates key components of Tai Chi that are central to Tai Chi's effectiveness for falls prevention. (2) It is straightforward to learn at a beginner level. (3) The movements can be readily modified so people with a wide range of medical issues and impairments can comfortably perform the exercises and benefit from them.

The benefits of practicing Tai Chi Circling Hands go well beyond avoiding falls. As an exercise, it delivers a powerful, low-impact workout for the entire body. For those interested in Qigong (energy practices) or Neigong (internal practices), Circling Hands provides an exceptional platform for deeply working the body and its energy.

To explore the many benefits of Tai Chi Circling Hands, I recommend the programs produced by Master Bruce Frantzis and his company, Energy Arts Inc. For more information, go to https://www.energyarts.com/.

---

Now, let's turn to Part 1 and start building the foundation for your Tai Chi for Balance practice.

# Part 1

# The Foundation:

# Before We Start Moving

The four chapters of Part 1 build the foundation for the Tai Chi for Balance System. In Chapter 1, we look at the hard facts of aging and falling and the hopeful science supporting fall prevention. Chapter 2 covers key concepts we apply throughout the program. In Chapter 3, we establish the Two Rules that guide all our activity in Tai Chi for Balance. In Chapter 4, we stand up and learn Neutral Posture, a specific way to align the body. From there, we begin to develop Whole Body Awareness by feeling our feet and center.

With that, turn to Chapter 1 and take your next step on the path to stability, security, and confidence on your feet.

# Chapter 1

# Aging and Falling: Bad News and Good News

This chapter covers key data on the risks of falling for older adults, the life-altering injuries that result, and the promising science on preventing falls. I include this information, grim as some of it seems, for three main reasons:

- **Knowledge can motivate change.** Research suggests that many older adults are *not* aware of the increased risks of falling.[1] Filling that knowledge gap will motivate you to make changes in your life to avoid falls. Changes like learning and practicing Tai Chi for Balance.
- **You can avoid falls.** A clear consensus exists among researchers and all leading medical authorities. ***Falls are preventable***.[2]
- **Tai Chi reduces your risk of falling.** Another clear consensus exists in the research. Exercise reduces falls risk.[3] One type of exercise consistently emerges as the most effective in reducing falls: Tai Chi.

First, let's look at the bad news.

---

[1] Judy A. Stevens, David A. Sleet, and Laurence Z. Rubenstein, "The Influence of Older Adults' Beliefs and Attitudes on Adopting Fall Prevention Behaviors," *American Journal of Lifestyle Medicine* 12, no. 4 (July 1, 2018): 324–30, https://doi.org/10.1177/1559827616687263.

[2] "CDC Compendium of Effective Fall Interventions: What Works for Community-Dwelling Older Adults, 3rd Edition | Home and Recreational Safety | CDC Injury Center," accessed November 23, 2016, http://www.cdc.gov/homeandrecreationalsafety/falls/compendium.html.

[3] Catherine Sherrington et al., "Exercise for Preventing Falls in Older People Living in the Community," *The Cochrane Database of Systematic Reviews* 1 (January 31, 2019): CD012424, https://doi.org/10.1002/14651858.CD012424.pub2.

# The Bad News: Older Adults and Falling

As we age, our risk of falling increases, especially at 65 years and up (65+). Falls data underscores the scope of the problem.

Annually in the US, among adults age 65+, about 1 in 3 falls.[1] For older adults, those falls:

- Are the #1 cause of injury.[2]
- Are the #1 cause of death from injury.[3]
- Send 3 million to the emergency room.[4]
- Result in more than 2.8 million injuries.[5]
- Put 800,000 in the hospital.[6]
- Cause about 30,000 deaths.[7]
- Incur more than $50 billion of total medical costs.[8]

---

[1] Sherrington et al.

[2] Gwen Bergen, Mark R. Stevens, and Elizabeth R. Burns, "Falls and Fall Injuries Among Adults Aged ≥65 Years - United States, 2014," *MMWR. Morbidity and Mortality Weekly Report* 65, no. 37 (September 23, 2016): 993–98, https://doi.org/10.15585/mmwr.mm6537a2.

[3] Bergen, Stevens, and Burns, "Falls and Fall Injuries," 993-98.

[4] "Facts About Falls | Fall Prevention | Injury Center | CDC," Centers for Disease Control and Prevention, December 1, 2021, https://www.cdc.gov/falls/facts.html.

[5] Bergen, Stevens, and Burns, "Falls and Fall Injuries," 993-98.

[6] Centers for Disease Control and Prevention, "Facts About Falls".

[7] Bergen, Stevens, and Burns, "Falls and Fall Injuries," 993-98.

[8] Curtis S. Florence et al., "Medical Costs of Fatal and Nonfatal Falls in Older Adults," *Journal of the American Geriatrics Society* 66, no. 4 (April 2018): 693–98, https://doi.org/10.1111/jgs.15304.

## Aging and Falling: Bad News and Good News

Let that sink in. Each year in the US, 3 million ER visits, 2.8 million injuries, 800,000 hospital admissions, 30,000 deaths, $50 billion in medical costs. All from falls.

It's no surprise that leading medical authorities recognize falling as a major health risk for older adults and a significant burden on our health care system.

But the bad news doesn't stop there. Consider the following:

- If you fall once, your risk of falling again doubles.[9]
- 1 out of 5 falls causes a serious injury, like a broken bone or head injury.[10]
- 300,000 older adults are hospitalized annually for broken hips. Falls cause more than 95% of broken hips.[11]
- About half of fallers who break a hip never functionally walk again.[12]
- 20% of fallers who break a hip die within 6 months.[13]

The serious injuries caused by falls have a heartbreaking consequence for older adults— **loss of independence**. Nearly two-thirds of older adults hospitalized for a

---

[9] Centers for Disease Control and Prevention, "Facts About Falls".

[10] Ibid.

[11] Ibid.

[12] "What Are the Main Risk Factors for Falls amongst Older People and What Are the Most Effective Interventions to Prevent These Falls?," Health Evidence Network, World Health Organization (2004), https://www.euro.who.int/__data/assets/pdf_file/0018/74700/E82552.pdf.

[13] World Health Organization, "What Are the Main Risk Factors for Falls amongst Older People?"

fall injury are later admitted to a long-term care facility.[14] Falls are a contributing factor to 40% of admissions to assisted living facilities.[15]

Falls threaten our mental and emotional health too. Falls contribute to depression, fear, loss of confidence, social withdrawal—even when there is no physical injury. Post-fall syndrome is a recognized psychological condition, characterized by fear of movement, loss of motivation, and loss of self-confidence.[16]

**Why do Older Adults Fall?**

Research suggests a range of factors increase the risk of falling as we age.[17] These include:

- Impaired mobility and gait
- Impaired balance
- Increased use of multiple medicines
- Declining health from chronic diseases
- Visual decline

---

[14] Geoffrey J. Hoffman et al., "The Costs of Fall-Related Injuries among Older Adults: Annual Per-Faller, Service Component, and Patient Out-of-Pocket Costs," *Health Services Research* 52, no. 5 (October 2017): 1794–1816, https://doi.org/10.1111/1475-6773.12554.

[15] World Health Organization, "What Are the Main Risk Factors for Falls amongst Older People?"

[16] Maxence Meyer et al., "Gait Disorder among Elderly People, Psychomotor Disadaptation Syndrome: Post-Fall Syndrome, Risk Factors and Follow-Up – A Cohort Study of 70 Patients," *Gerontology* 67, no. 1 (2021): 17–24, https://doi.org/10.1159/000511356.

[17] World Health Organization, "What Are the Main Risk Factors for Falls amongst Older People?"; Silvia Deandrea et al., "Risk Factors for Falls in Community-Dwelling Older People: A Systematic Review and Meta-Analysis," *Epidemiology (Cambridge, Mass.)* 21, no. 5 (September 2010): 658–68, https://doi.org/10.1097/EDE.0b013e3181e89905; Edward W. Gregg, Mark A. Pereira, and Carl J. Caspersen, "Physical Activity, Falls, and Fractures Among Older Adults: A Review of the Epidemiologic Evidence," *Journal of the American Geriatrics Society* 48, no. 8 (2000): 883–93, https://doi.org/10.1111/j.1532-5415.2000.tb06884.x; Lida Hosseini et al., "Tai Chi Chuan Can Improve Balance and Reduce Fear of Falling in Community Dwelling Older Adults: A Randomized Control Trial," *Journal of Exercise Rehabilitation* 14, no. 6 (December 2018): 1024–31, https://doi.org/10.12965/jer.1836488.244.

- Cognitive impairment

In short, age-related declines in health and physical function increase the risk of falling. We can mitigate these risks to a degree. For example, we can update our eyeglass prescription. We can work with a physician on managing multiple medicines. We can maintain treatment plans for chronic diseases. That said, the body changes as we age, and we have limited ability to reverse many of those changes.

Research suggests the #1 risk factor for falling is **lower extremity muscle weakness.**[18] This means loss of strength in the legs and hips. Loss of muscle mass, called sarcopenia, occurs with age. Maintaining balance and recovering from a loss of balance requires muscles throughout the body, especially in the hips and legs, to generate force. If the muscles weaken and cannot generate sufficient force to stabilize us, we're more likely to fall.

Unlike many age-related risks factors, we counteract age-related muscle weakness. How? ***Exercise***.

We'll turn to that shortly.

The data about aging and falling may seem grim, but I share it to arm you with knowledge. That knowledge can motivate positive change, inspiring you to take steps to reduce the risk of falling.

Ready for some good news? Let's turn to that now.

---

[18] Vicky Scott PhD, *Fall Prevention Programming: Designing, Implementing and Evaluating Fall Prevention Programs for Older Adults*, Second Edition (Vancouver: Dr. Vicky Scott, 2017); Julie D. Moreland et al., "Muscle Weakness and Falls in Older Adults: A Systematic Review and Meta-Analysis," *Journal of the American Geriatrics Society* 52, no. 7 (July 2004): 1121–29, https://doi.org/10.1111/j.1532-5415.2004.52310.x.

# The Good News: Falls are Preventable

Leading medical authorities agree—*we can prevent falls*. The CDC, "We know that falls are not an inevitable cause of aging. Prevention interventions reduce falls."[19]

Leading to a question: What are falls prevention interventions?

Extensive research has focused on this question. The answer emerging from that research is this: "Exercises that target balance, gait, and muscle strength have been found to prevent falls."[20] Because of that research, all leading medical authorities recommend *exercise* for preventing falls.

Leading to another question: What exercise should we do?

Here's how leading medical authorities answer that question:

### Centers for Disease Control

"Do exercises that make your legs stronger and improve your balance. *Tai Chi is a good example of this kind of exercise.*"[21]

### World Health Organization

"*Tai Chi is likely to be effective in preventing falls.*"[22]

### Harvard Medical School

---

[19] "CDC Compendium of Effective Fall Interventions: What Works for Community-Dwelling Older Adults, 3rd Edition | Home and Recreational Safety | CDC Injury Center."

[20] Sherrington et al., "Exercise for Preventing Falls in Older People Living in the Community."

[21] Centers for Disease Control and Prevention, "Facts About Falls."

[22] World Health Organization, "What Are the Main Risk Factors for Falls amongst Older People?"

"There's very strong evidence that *Tai Chi is one of the best weight-bearing exercises to reduce the risk for falls.*"[23]

**Mayo Clinic**

"*Only one [exercise] has actually been shown to prevent falls, and it's Tai Chi.*"[24]

**National Institutes of Health, National Center for Complementary and Integrative Care**

"*Tai Chi may be beneficial in improving balance and preventing falls in older adults…*"[25]

Notice the consistent response? They all recommend Tai Chi for falls prevention.

Why? **The science.**

# The Science: Tai Chi and Falls Prevention

Extensive research provides strong evidence that Tai Chi practice reduces falls in older adults. In this section, I describe a sample of that research.

If you're interested in exploring more of the research into Tai Chi for falls prevention, I include a list of research articles and other resources at the end of this chapter.

**Tai Chi and Falls Prevention: 2020 Analysis of the Evidence**

---

[23] "Protect Your Bones with Tai Chi," Harvard Health, October 1, 2020, https://www.health.harvard.edu/womens-health/protect-your-bones-with-tai-chi.

[24] "Mayo Clinic Minute: Tai Chi Keeps Seniors on Their Feet," Mayo Clinic News Network, April 2, 2018, https://newsnetwork.mayoclinic.org/discussion/mayo-clinic-minute-tai-chi-keeps-seniors-on-their-feet/.

[25] "Tai Chi: What Your Need to Know," National Center for Complementary and Integrative Health, https://www.nccih.nih.gov/health/tai-chi-what-you-need-to-know.

I begin with a 2020 article by Dr. Samuel Nyman, "Tai Chi for the Prevention of Falls Among Older Adults: A Critical Analysis of the Evidence,"[26] In this article, Dr. Nyman reviews the existing "gold-standard evidence" on Tai Chi and falls prevention: **meta-analyses of random controlled trials**.

To clarify what that means, a **random controlled trial** is a study that randomly assigns subjects to two or more groups. One group is the intervention group—for example, participating in 24 weeks of Tai Chi training. The other group is the control group. The control group doesn't participate in the intervention. Researchers take measurements before and after the intervention period, like number of falls, leg strength, and clinical tests of balance and falls risks. Then they statistically analyze differences in the data between the groups after the intervention period.

If a meaningful difference emerges—for example, the Tai Chi group has significantly fewer falls or significantly improved balance tests compared to the control group, then that provides evidence that the intervention, Tai Chi, caused the improvement.

So that's a **random controlled trial**.

A **meta-analysis** involves analysis of multiple random controlled trials. It's a study of multiple studies. Using sophisticated statistical techniques, a meta-analysis evaluates results from multiple studies, benefiting from a larger pool of subjects and a larger body of data.

Back to Dr. Nyman's article. He reviewed seven meta-analyses of Tai Chi as an intervention for falls prevention. **Those meta-analyses concluded that Tai Chi training significantly reduced falls, with reductions in fall rates ranging from 20% to 58%.**[27]

Dr. Nyman also examined several studies evaluating how Tai Chi compared to other exercises in preventing falls. These include studies comparing Tai Chi to computerized

---

[26] Samuel R. Nyman, "Tai Chi for the Prevention of Falls Among Older Adults: A Critical Analysis of the Evidence," *Journal of Aging and Physical Activity* 29, no. 2 (August 24, 2020): 343–52, https://doi.org/10.1123/japa.2020-0155.

[27] Ibid.

balance training, yoga, physical therapy, aerobic exercise, lower-extremity exercise, and multi-modal exercise (MME). (MME combines moderate aerobic exercise and light resistance exercise.) **The studies consistently showed that Tai Chi improved their balance and reduced falls more than any other exercise.**

Dr. Nyman's article emphasizes another key point in considering falls prevention exercises: **Tai Chi is safe.** He writes, "[O]ver 500 trials and 120 systematic reviews have been conducted on the health benefits of Tai Chi and no studies have found that Tai Chi worsens a condition."[28]

From this evidence, Dr. Nyman concludes:

> **"Tai Chi can be highly effective for preventing falls. Tai Chi is a safe and accessible form of exercise."** [29]

From Dr. Nyman's comprehensive analysis, I'll drill down into two specific studies.

**Tai Chi and Falls Prevention: The Most Effective Exercise**

Next, let's consider an important study evaluating how Tai Chi compares to other exercises for falls prevention. Reported in 2018 in the *Journal of the American Medical Association*, the study evaluated three exercise types: Tai Chi, MME, and stretching.[30]

670 subjects participated in the study, with a mean age of 78. Subjects were randomly assigned to one of the three interventions. They then participated in 60 minutes classes, twice per week for 24 weeks. Before and after the intervention, researchers collected data on falls history and clinical measures of balance.

---

[28] Ibid.

[29] Ibid.

[30] Fuzhong Li et al., "Effectiveness of a Therapeutic Tai Ji Quan Intervention vs a Multimodal Exercise Intervention to Prevent Falls Among Older Adults at High Risk of Falling: A Randomized Clinical Trial," *JAMA Internal Medicine* 178, no. 10 (October 1, 2018): 1301–10, https://doi.org/10.1001/jamainternmed.2018.3915.

The outcome? **The Tai Chi group experienced significantly fewer falls than both the MME group and the stretching group**. Strong evidence pointing to Tai Chi's effectiveness at preventing falls.

The next study considers a key aspect of falls prevention interventions, the cost.

**Tai Chi and Falls Prevention: The Most Cost-Effective Intervention**

In evaluating risk reduction interventions, especially for a major medical issue like falling, cost presents an important issue. Higher cost interventions create barriers to implementation and participation. Conversely, an intervention providing a significant reduction in falls at a low cost reduces the financial burden on sponsoring organizations and participants, lowering barriers to implementation and participation.

Research suggests the most cost-effective falls prevention intervention is Tai Chi.

A study reported in 2015 conducted a cost-benefit analysis of three falls prevention programs. The programs studied were the Otago Exercise Program, Stepping On, and a Tai Chi-based program.[31]

The researchers estimated the implementation costs of each program, the average medical costs of falls-related injuries, and the resultant savings from the reduction in falls among program participants. From this, the study derived a return on investment (ROI) for each program.

The researchers found that each of the programs reduced falls among the participants and saved money by reducing medical costs. So each of the programs had a positive ROI. The study calculated the Otago Exercise Program ROI at 144%, and the Stepping On ROI at 64%.

---

[31] Vilma Carande-Kulis et al., "A Cost-Benefit Analysis of Three Older Adult Fall Prevention Interventions," *Journal of Safety Research* 52 (February 2015): 65–70, https://doi.org/10.1016/j.jsr.2014.12.007.

Of the three programs, the Tai Chi program was overwhelmingly the most cost-effective, delivering an ROI of a whopping **509%.** This means that each dollar spent on the Tai Chi program saved more than $5 in medical costs.

In short, when it comes to fall prevention, Tai Chi delivers the biggest bang for your buck.

**Tai Chi and Falls Prevention: Directions for Future Research**

Current science provides strong evidence supporting Tai Chi as the most effective exercise-based falls prevention program. Still, lots of questions remain.

For example, what elements of Tai Chi training contribute most to falls prevention? Conversely, what aspects of Tai Chi training do not contribute to falls prevention? Answers to these questions will help us better tailor falls prevention programs emphasizing the most effective elements of Tai Chi.

Science is a process. A dynamic, imperfect, and, at times, contentious process. That process continually builds upon, corrects, sometimes refutes, and most often evolves from the current scientific understanding of our world.

For our purposes, the most important point of the current scientific understanding of our world is this: **As we age, Tai Chi training will help us stay on our feet and avoid falls.**

With that background, let's turn to the next chapter and explore *key concepts* underlying the Tai Chi for Balance System.

# Chapter Wrap-Up

This chapter presents the bad news and good news about aging and falling. Key takeaways include:

**Older Adults and Falling— A Major Threat to Health and Independence**

- The risk of injury from falling begins to increase at about age 60.
- By age 65, falling is the #1 cause of injury and death from injury.
- 1 out of 5 falls causes a serious injury, like a broken bone or head injury.
- Nearly two-thirds of older adults hospitalized for a fall injury are later admitted to long-term care.
- Falling is a contributing factor in 40% of admissions to assisted living facilities.

To maintain our health and independence, we want to stay on our feet and avoid falls.

**Falls Risk Factors**

- A major risk factor for falling is **lower extremity muscle weakness**. Strengthening the legs and hips with exercises like Tai Chi mitigates this risk factor.
- Other risk factors include:
    - Visual decline
    - Impaired mobility and gait
    - Impaired balance
    - Increased use of multiple medicines
    - Declining health from chronic diseases
    - Cognitive impairment

**Falls Are Preventable**

- Leading medical authorities agree: Falls are preventable.

**Tai Chi Is the Most Effective and Cost-Effective Exercise for Reducing Falls**

Research shows:

- Older adults participating in Tai Chi training fall significantly less.
- Tai Chi training reduces falls more than other types of exercise training.
- Tai Chi is the most cost-effective falls prevention intervention.

# Studies Evaluating Tai Chi as an Intervention for Falls Prevention and Other Resources.

Chodzko-Zajko, Wojtek J., David N. Proctor, Maria A. Fiatarone Singh, Christopher T. Minson, Claudio R. Nigg, George J. Salem, and James S. Skinner. "Exercise and Physical Activity for Older Adults." *Medicine & Science in Sports & Exercise* 41, no. 7 (July 2009): 1510–30. https://doi.org/10.1249/MSS.0b013e3181a0c95c.

Centers for Disease Control and Prevention, "Facts About Falls | Fall Prevention | Injury Center | CDC," December 1, 2021. https://www.cdc.gov/falls/facts.html.

Fuzhong Li, Peter Harmer, Karin A. Mack, David Sleet, K. John Fisher, Melvin A. Kohn, Lisa M. Millet, et al. "Tai Chi: Moving for Better Balance-Development of a Community-Based Falls Prevention Program." *Journal of Physical Activity & Health* 5, no. 3 (May 2008): 445–55. https://doi.org/10.1123/jpah.5.3.445.

Gallant, Mary P., Meaghan Tartaglia, Susan Hardman, and Kara Burke. "Using Tai Chi to Reduce Fall Risk Factors Among Older Adults: An Evaluation of a Community-Based Implementation." *Journal of Applied Gerontology* 38, no. 7 (July 2019): 983–98. https://doi.org/10.1177/0733464817703004.

Gregg, Edward W., Mark A. Pereira, and Carl J. Caspersen. "Physical Activity, Falls, and Fractures Among Older Adults: A Review of the Epidemiologic Evidence." *Journal of the American Geriatrics Society* 48, no. 8 (August 2000): 883–93. https://doi.org/10.1111/j.1532-5415.2000.tb06884.x.

Hosseini, Lida, Elham Kargozar, Farshad Sharifi, Reza Negarandeh, Amir-Hossein Memari, and Elham Navab. "Tai Chi Chuan Can Improve Balance and Reduce Fear of Falling in Community Dwelling Older Adults: A Randomized Control Trial." *Journal of Exercise Rehabilitation* 14, no. 6 (December 2018): 1024–31. https://doi.org/10.12965/jer.1836488.244.

Huang, Zhi-Guan, Yun-Hui Feng, Yu-He Li, and Chang-Sheng Lv. "Systematic Review and Meta-Analysis: Tai Chi for Preventing Falls in Older Adults." *BMJ Open* 7, no. 2 (February 6, 2017): e013661. https://doi.org/10.1136/bmjopen-2016-013661.

Kim J, Foucher K. "Fall experiences from the perspectives of people with osteoarthritis: in their own words." Disabil Rehabil. 2022 Dec 15:1-9. https://pubmed.ncbi.nlm.nih.gov/36519505/

Li, Fuzhong. "The Effects of Tai Ji Quan Training on Limits of Stability in Older Adults." *Clinical Interventions in Aging* 9 (2014): 1261–68. https://doi.org/10.2147/CIA.S65823.

Li, Fuzhong. "Transforming Traditional Tai Ji Quan Techniques into Integrative Movement Therapy-Tai Ji Quan: Moving for Better *Balance*." *Journal of Sport and Health Science* 3, no. 1 (March 1, 2014): 9–15. https://doi.org/10.1016/j.jshs.2013.11.002.

Li, Fuzhong, Elizabeth Eckstrom, Peter Harmer, Kathleen Fitzgerald, Jan Voit, and Kathleen A. Cameron. "Exercise and Fall Prevention: Narrowing the Research-to-Practice Gap and Enhancing Integration of Clinical and Community Practice." *Journal of the American Geriatrics Society* 64, no. 2 (February 2016): 425–31. https://doi.org/10.1111/jgs.13925.

Li, Fuzhong, Peter Harmer, Elizabeth Eckstrom, Kathleen Fitzgerald, Li-Shan Chou, and Yu Liu. "Effectiveness of Tai Ji Quan vs Multimodal and Stretching Exercise Interventions for Reducing Injurious Falls in Older Adults at High Risk of Falling: Follow-up Analysis of a Randomized Clinical Trial." *JAMA Network Open* 2, no. 2 (February 15, 2019): e188280. https://doi.org/10.1001/jamanetworkopen.2018.8280.

Li, Fuzhong, Peter Harmer, K. John Fisher, and Edward McAuley. "Tai Chi: Improving Functional Balance and Predicting Subsequent Falls in Older Persons." *Medicine and Science in Sports and Exercise* 36, no. 12 (December 2004): 2046–52.

Li, Fuzhong, Peter Harmer, K. John Fisher, Edward McAuley, Nigel Chaumeton, Elizabeth Eckstrom, and Nicole L. Wilson. "Tai Chi and Fall Reductions in Older Adults: A Randomized Controlled Trial." *The Journals of Gerontology. Series A, Biological Sciences and Medical Sciences* 60, no. 2 (February 2005): 187–94. https://doi.org/10.1093/gerona/60.2.187.

Li, Fuzhong, Peter Harmer, and Kathleen Fitzgerald. "Implementing an Evidence-Based Fall Prevention Intervention in Community Senior Centers." *American Journal of Public Health* 106, no. 11 (November 2016): 2026–31. https://doi.org/10.2105/AJPH.2016.303386.

Li, Fuzhong, Peter Harmer, Russell Glasgow, Karin A. Mack, David Sleet, K. John Fisher, Melvin A. Kohn, et al. "Translation of an Effective Tai Chi Intervention into a Community-Based Falls-Prevention Program." *American Journal of Public Health* 98, no. 7 (July 2008): 1195–98. https://doi.org/10.2105/AJPH.2007.120402.

Li, Fuzhong, Peter Harmer, Ronald Stock, Kathleen Fitzgerald, Judy Stevens, Michele Gladieux, Li-Shan Chou, Kenji Carp, and Jan Voit. "Implementing an Evidence-Based Fall Prevention Program in an Outpatient Clinical Setting." *Journal of the American Geriatrics Society* 61, no. 12 (December 1, 2013): 2142–49. https://doi.org/10.1111/jgs.12509.

Lomas-Vega, Rafael, Esteban Obrero-Gaitán, Francisco J. Molina-Ortega, and Rafael Del-Pino-Casado. "Tai Chi for Risk of Falls. A Meta-Analysis." *Journal of the American Geriatrics Society* 65, no. 9 (September 2017): 2037–43. https://doi.org/10.1111/jgs.15008.

Mayo Clinic News Network. "Mayo Clinic Minute: Tai Chi Keeps Seniors on Their Feet," April 2, 2018. https://newsnetwork.mayoclinic.org/discussion/mayo-clinic-minute-tai-chi-keeps-seniors-on-their-feet/.

Nyman, Samuel R. "Tai Chi for the Prevention of Falls Among Older Adults: A Critical Analysis of the Evidence." *Journal of Aging and Physical Activity* 29, no. 2 (August 24, 2020): 343–52. https://doi.org/10.1123/japa.2020-0155.

Ory, Marcia G., Matthew Lee Smith, Erin M. Parker, Luohua Jiang, Shuai Chen, Ashley D. Wilson, Judy A. Stevens, Heidi Ehrenreich, and Robin Lee. "Fall Prevention in Community Settings: Results from Implementing Tai Chi: Moving for Better Balance in Three States." *Frontiers in Public Health* 2 (2014): 258. https://doi.org/10.3389/fpubh.2014.00258.

Penn, I.-Wen, Wen-Hsu Sung, Chien-Hui Lin, Eric Chuang, Tien-Yow Chuang, and Pei-Hsin Lin. "Effects of Individualized Tai-Chi on Balance and Lower-Limb Strength in Older Adults." *BMC Geriatrics* 19, no. 1 (August 27, 2019): 235. https://doi.org/10.1186/s12877-019-1250-8.

Sherrington, Catherine, Nicola J. Fairhall, Geraldine K. Wallbank, Anne Tiedemann, Zoe A Michaleff, Kirsten Howard, Lindy Clemson, Sally Hopewell, and Sarah E Lamb. "Exercise for Preventing Falls in Older People Living in the Community." *The Cochrane Database of Systematic Reviews* 2019, no. 1 (January 31, 2019): CD012424. https://doi.org/10.1002/14651858.CD012424.pub2.

World Health Organization. "What Are the Main Risk Factors for Falls amongst Older People and What Are the Most Effective Interventions to Prevent These Falls?" Health Evidence Network, (2004), https://www.euro.who.int/__data/assets/pdf_file/0018/74700/E82552.pdf.

Zhong, Dongling, Qiwei Xiao, Xili Xiao, Yuxi Li, Jing Ye, Lina Xia, Chi Zhang, Juan Li, Hui Zheng, and Rongjiang Jin. "Tai Chi for Improving Balance and Reducing Falls: An Overview of 14 Systematic Reviews." *Annals of Physical and Rehabilitation Medicine* 63, no. 6 (November 2020): 505–17. https://doi.org/10.1016/j.rehab.2019.12.008.

# Chapter 2

# Key Concepts

This chapter introduces key concepts incorporated throughout Tai Chi for Balance. These include:

- Stability
- Center of gravity
- Base of support
- How to increase stability
- Whole Body Awareness
- Precise Posture Control

By the end of this chapter, you'll have a practical understanding of these key concepts and why they're important for staying on your feet and avoiding falls.

## Stability

**Why *Stability* Is More Important Than *Balance* for Avoiding Falls**

Note I do not identify "balance" as a key concept. Why's that?

My position: **For avoiding falls, *stability* is more important than balance**.

That's right. From years of study, training, teaching, and observing, I conclude that to prevent falls, training that develops *greater stability* is more important than training that improves measures of balance.

To understand why, let's start by defining these terms.

## What Is "Balance"?

According to Merriam-Webster's dictionary, "balance" means "physical equilibrium," with weight evenly distributed about a vertical axis.[1] In this sense, balance is a *static state*.

Imagine a gymnast standing on one leg on a 4-inch-wide beam several feet above the floor. That requires physical equilibrium, or balance.

## What Is "Stability"?

In contrast, consider the definition of "stability":

> "Stability is the capacity of an object [including a human] to return to equilibrium or to its original position after it has been displaced."[2]

Stability determines our ability to **return to equilibrium after being displaced**. From this definition, we see stability has a ***dynamic*** quality to it.

For "being displaced," we can substitute words and phrases like "slipping," "tripping," "bumped in a crowd," or "yanked by the dog." Stability governs our ability to avoid a fall from these and other disturbances to our equilibrium. The more stable we are, the more likely we are to return to equilibrium after something knocks us off equilibrium.

It also helps to keep our #1 objective in mind— Staying on your feet and avoiding falls. Our aim is to step, walk, stroll, ambulate, and navigate our world on two feet—all while *avoiding unintended trips to the ground.*

To do that, **our training needs to focus on increasing *stability***. By following the Tai Chi for Balance System, you'll develop the sensitivity and skills needed to maintain an increasingly stable structure through increasingly dynamic movement.

---

[1] "Balance," Merriam-Webster Dictionary, accessed April 2023, https://www.merriam-webster.com/dictionary/balance.

[2] Peter M. McGinnis, *Biomechanics of Sport and Exercise*, 4th edition (Human Kinetics, 2020), Kindle.

*Key Concepts*

The remaining key concepts link directly to stability.

# Center of Gravity

Center of gravity, also called center of mass, is defined as follows:

> "The point in a body around which its weight is evenly distributed and through which the force of gravity acts."[3]

That seems like a mouthful, I recognize. Grab a pencil and let's try a practical example.

Extend one index finger and place the pencil across your finger. Then adjust it until it balances on your finger. (Figure 2-1.)

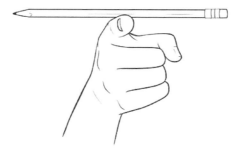

*Figure 2-1: Balancing a pencil. Is it stable?*

Your finger is now under the center of gravity of the pencil. Its weight is evenly distributed around that point, and gravity acts on the pencil through that point.

You could also say the pencil has reached a state of equilibrium. It's balanced across your finger. So long as no other force displaces the object, it will stay in that state of equilibrium. The pencil is balanced. But is it stable? Let's see.

With your other index finger, apply a light force to the end of the pencil. What happens? (Figure 2-2.)

---

[3] Ibid.

# TAI CHI FOR BALANCE

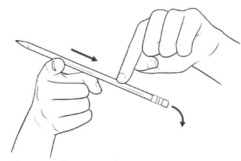

*Figure 2-2: A force displacing the pencil.*

In most cases, the pencil falls off your finger. It doesn't return to equilibrium. We can conclude the object is not stable.

An important point about center of gravity when it comes to humans: Humans have moving parts. Lots of them. When you move any of your parts, you can change your center of gravity.

For example, when standing as shown in Figure 2-3A, our center of gravity is slightly below the navel in the center of our body.

Then, if we lean to the side, our center of gravity moves some distance in that direction. (Figure 2-3B.)

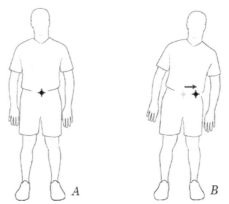

*Figure 2-3: Leaning to the side moves our center of gravity to the side.*

## Key Concepts

Similarly, let's consider the profile view of a person standing in a vertical posture. (Figure 2-4A.) In this position, the center of gravity is in the center of the body, slightly below the navel.

Next, let's bring the head forward and collapse the posture forward a little. (Figure 2-4B.)

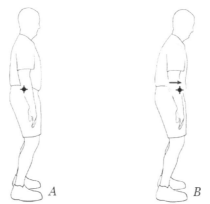

*Figure 2-4: Leaning forward moves our center of gravity forward.*

This moves the center of gravity forward.

As we'll explore later in this chapter, the location of your center of gravity directly affects your stability. In Tai Chi for Balance, you'll gain skill at controlling your center of gravity to increase stability, mainly through developing Precise Posture Control.

## Base of Support

In biomechanics, we define "**base of support**" as:

> "The area beneath and between the points of contact an object has with the ground."[4]

---

[4] Ibid.

To illustrate this concept, let's consider a book. Assume the book is 10 inches tall, 10 inches wide, and 1 inch thick. (Figure 2-5.)

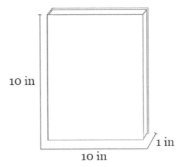

*Figure 2-5*

If we stand the book on edge, we can calculate the base of support as 10 inches x 1 inch = 10 inches squared. (Figure 2-6A.)

If we lay the book on its cover, we can calculate the base of support as 10 inches x 10 inches = 100 inches squared. (Figure 2-6B.)

In which position is the book more stable? That is, less prone to toppling over if displaced?

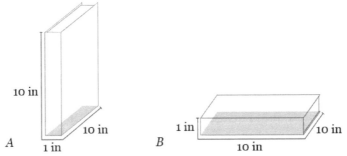

*Figure 2-6: Increasing the book's base of support makes it more stable.*

There's no question; position B is more stable than position A. We know this intuitively. But why? **A larger base of support makes an object more stable.**

## Key Concepts

Next, let's apply that key concept to a type of object especially relevant to Tai Chi for Balance—a human.

Consider two positions in which we can place our bodies. (Figure 2-7A and B.)

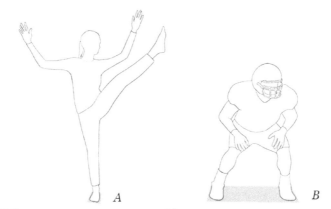

Figure 2-7: What position is more stable?

The shaded area shows the base of support. Which position is more stable, that is, less prone to toppling over if pushed?

Again, there's no question that the person in position B is more stable. By establishing a larger base of support, the person is less likely to topple over if pushed.

With this understanding of center of gravity and base of support, let's explore how to increase stability.

## How to Increase Stability

This key concept goes to the heart of what we're up to in Tai Chi for Balance, increasing stability so you become resistant to falling.

Here's how you do it:

**You increase your stability by managing your center of gravity and your base of support.**

More specifically, you can increase stability by managing your center of gravity and base of support in three distinct ways:

1. You increase stability by increasing your base of support.

2. You increase stability by maintaining your center of gravity closer to the center of your base of support.

3. You increase stability by lowering your center of gravity.

To get a handle on these ideas, let's consider two iconic structures: the exquisite Mayan pyramid at Chichen Itza and the elegant Leaning Tower of Pisa. (Figures 2-8A and B.)

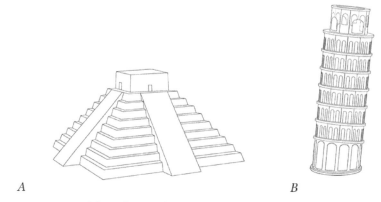

*Figure 2-8: Pyramid and Leaning Tower.*

Which structure is more stable? That is, which structure is harder to knock over? In about one second, we answer, "Obviously, the pyramid!"

But why? Several reasons, which we cover in the next sections.

*Key Concepts*

## The Size of the Base of Support

First, let's consider the respective bases of support. (Figure 2-9A-B.)

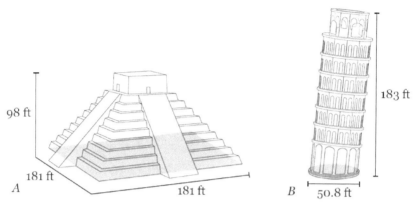

*Figure 2-9: Pyramid and Leaning Tower, comparing bases of support.*

Here, we can see that the pyramid's base of support is larger than the Leaning Tower's. We can also calculate the square footage of the respective bases of support.

Pyramid: 181 ft x 181 ft = 32,761 ft²

Leaning Tower: (½ 50.8 ft)² x π = 2025 ft²

That larger base of support contributes to the pyramid's greater stability. Conversely, because the Leaning Tower has a smaller base of support, it's less stable.

## Location of the Center of Gravity within the Base of Support

Next, let's consider the locations of the respective centers of gravity within each structure's base of support.

Note how the pyramid's center of gravity falls within the center of its base of support. (Figure 2-10A.)

In contrast, because the Tower of Pisa leans, its center of gravity is closer to the edge of its base of support. (Figure 2-10B.)

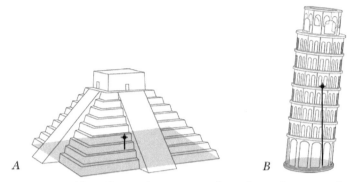

*Figure 2-10: Pyramid and Leaning Tower, location of center of gravity in relation to base of support.*

Because the pyramid's center of gravity is closer to the center of its base of support, the structure is more stable, less likely to topple. Conversely, because the Leaning Tower's center of gravity falls closer to the edge of its base of support, it's less stable and more likely to topple.

**Height of Center of Gravity**

Next, let's consider the height of the structures' respective centers of gravity.

Note how the pyramid's mass is concentrated in the lower part of the structure. This lowers the center of gravity. (Figure 2-11A.)

Note how the Leaning Tower's mass is more evenly distributed through the upper and lower parts of the structure. This raises its center of gravity. (Figure 2-11B.)

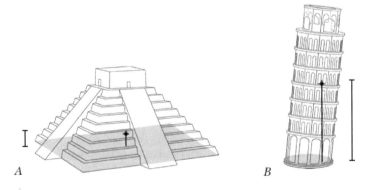

*Figure 2-11: Pyramid and Leaning Tower, height of center of gravity.*

Because the pyramid's center of gravity is lower, it's more stable and less likely to topple. And because the Leaning Tower's center of gravity is higher, it's less stable and more likely to topple.

**Why the Pyramid is More Stable than the Leaning Tower**

By looking at the two structures, we intuitively know the pyramid is more stable than the Leaning Tower. Now we have concepts and language to articulate why. We can say, compared to the Leaning Tower, the pyramid is more stable because:

- It has a larger base of support.
- Its center of gravity is closer to the center of its base of support.
- Its center of gravity is lower.

Conversely, we can say, compared to the pyramid, the Leaning Tower is less stable because:

- It has a smaller base of support.
- Its center of gravity is closer to the edge of its base of support.
- Its center of gravity is higher.

**So what? I'm not a building!**

At this point, you might think, "So what? I'm not a pyramid or Leaning Tower!"

Fair point. But consider this: You, me, and all humans are *structures*, subject to the same mechanical forces as buildings.

Let's now consider a human structure. In this case, mine!

# TAI CHI FOR BALANCE

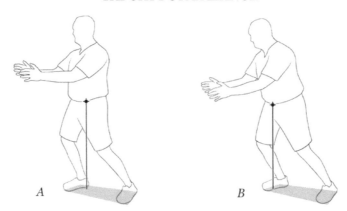

*Figure 2-12: What position is less stable? Why?*

Figure 2-12 depicts me performing one of the movements you'll learn soon, Vertical Circles + Weight Shift. I've shifted my weight to the front leg and circled my arms and hands to the front of my Vertical Circle.

In Figure 2-12A, my posture is vertical. Note how my center of gravity is more toward the center of my base of support.

In Figure 2-12B, I'm leaning. For people who have not received Tai Chi for Balance training, it's common to lean when shifting weight. Even more so when extending the arms. Note how my center of gravity falls close to the edge of my base of support. Consequently, I am less stable. Holding this position, a little push from behind could send me toppling forward. (Figure 2-13.)

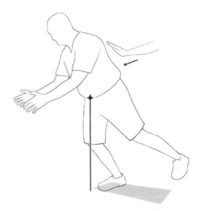

*Figure 2-13: From a less stable position to toppling over.*

**The Big Point: Learning How to Maintain a More Stable Structure**

I share these key concepts with you for one main reason: In my experience, people appreciate and benefit from an understanding of fundamental concepts of stability. As we proceed through the Tai Chi for Balance program, you will get plenty of practice applying these key concepts to develop a more stable structure.

# Whole Body Awareness

Developing a more stable structure requires that we feel our bodies. That leads to the next key concept— **Whole Body Awareness**.

For example, we need to feel our feet. That helps us develop a more stable base of support. Consistently feeling our feet also helps us feel the walking surface below them, changes to that surface, and obstacles contacting our feet—all very helpful information for avoiding falls.

We also need to feel where our head, torso, and arms are in relation to our hips, legs, and feet. This helps us maintain our center of gravity more toward the center of our base of support.

In developing Whole Body Awareness, we encounter a problem. In our society, people spend nearly all their time with their minds in their heads. Most, if not all, of our education focuses on developing the ability to think. Manipulating symbols, like letters and numbers. Analyzing information. Solving problems. All of which happens in our heads.

We receive little, if any, training in developing sensitivity to the sensations produced by our bodies. Like the sense of *proprioception*, the ability to feel where parts of the body are in space and in relation to each other. Or the sense of *interoception*, the ability to feel inside the body.

Tai Chi for Balance will help you fill in the blanks in that education. You'll learn and practice Whole Body Awareness, contributing to maintaining a more stable, fall-resistant structure. Two areas of the body we'll focus on a lot are **your feet** and **your center**.

## **Precise Posture Control**

The final key concept is Precise Posture Control.

As our comparison of the pyramid and the Leaning Tower demonstrates, a more upright, vertical posture creates a more stable structure. Why?

We know how to answer that question now: A more upright, vertical posture positions our center of gravity closer to the center of our base of support, making us less susceptible to toppling over.

The problem is most people do not maintain a vertical posture. They tend to lean. Watch people stand and walk, especially older adults. You'll see lots of leaning. This results in a less stable structure and greater susceptibility to falling.

In Tai Chi for Balance, you'll learn how to control your posture with increasing precision. You'll position your body in a relaxed, upright, vertical posture. First while standing. Then while performing increasingly dynamic movements.

One way to think about it is this: You'll become more like the pyramid and less like the Leaning Tower.

That completes the introduction of our key concepts. For the Two Rules governing all that you'll do in the Tai Chi for Balance System, turn to the next chapter.

# Chapter Wrap-Up

This chapter covered key concepts we'll apply throughout Tai Chi for Balance. Here's a recap of main points.

**For Avoiding Falls, Stability Is More Important than Balance**

Balance means *static equilibrium*. Stability means the ability to return to equilibrium after being displaced. Most falls occur when we experience a "displacement"—a slip, trip, bump, or other destabilizing force. To avoid a fall, we need to return to equilibrium. Greater stability is the key to that.

**Center of Gravity**

Center of gravity is an imaginary point in a body around which the weight is evenly distributed and through which gravity acts. Awareness and control of your center of gravity is key to developing a more stable structure.

**Base of Support**

Base of support means the area beneath and between where you contact the ground. Awareness and control of your base of support provides another key to developing a more stable structure.

**How to Increase Your Stability**

You can increase stability in three distinct ways: (i) Increasing your base of support, (ii) positioning your center of gravity closer to the center of your base of support, and (iii) lowering your center of gravity.

**Whole Body Awareness**

Our sense of proprioception enables us to feel where our body is in space. Our sense of interoception enables us to feel inside our bodies. Feeling more of your body is key to maintaining a more stable structure.

**Precise Posture Control**

A more upright, vertical posture contributes to maintaining a more stable structure. We want to be more like the pyramid and less like the Leaning Tower.

# Chapter 3

# The Two Rules

This chapter covers the Two Rules governing Tai Chi for Balance. The Two Rules apply to all the material you'll learn and practice in this program.

The Two Rules are straightforward. But for many of us, *these rules conflict with a lifetime of conditioning.* We are not used to feeling and caring for our bodies in the ways I'm about to describe.

For most of us, it takes a little effort (and a few reminders) to adapt to these rules. I assure you this: Your effort will be richly rewarded. By following the Two Rules, you'll accelerate your progress toward feeling stable, secure, and confident on your feet. You may experience powerfully positive change in other areas of your life too.

## Rule #1: The 70% Rule

The 70% Rule holds:

> **In Tai Chi for Balance, we perform all movements and all practices to no more than 70% of our maximum.**

For those of us who have spent years driving ourselves to "give 110%," the 70% Rule sounds bizarre. You might think, "How can I succeed at anything without pushing, striving, or straining?"

From the perspective of Tai Chi—a sophisticated, time-tested practice that promotes health, healing, and longevity—the 70% Rule makes complete sense. Here are two main reasons why.

- **The 70% Rule promotes relaxation and healing.** In Tai Chi, we aim to relax the body at ever deeper levels. At a range of motion that is 70% of your maximum, you increase your ability to move *and* relax. This leads to many positive consequences for health and healing, including reduction in chronic tension, increased mobility, and improved blood circulation.
- **The 70% Rule reduces the risk of injury.** In Tai Chi, we aim to heal the body, not hurt it. The closer we get to 100% of our range of motion, or to 100% of our maximum volume of practice, the closer we get to *beyond* 100%. When we go beyond our 100%, we face a greater likelihood of injury.

**Feel How the 70% Rule Works**

Here's a quick exercise to feel the 70% Rule in action.

Lift both arms to approximately shoulder height, with your hands in front of you, palms facing the floor. Then extend your arms and hands straight out until you feel you are near 100% of your ability to extend. (Figure 3-1A.) Feel your shoulders. Are they tense, tight, hiked up toward your ears? Feel your elbows, hands and fingers. Are they tense?

Next, reduce the extension of your arms to approximately 70% of your maximum. (Figure 3-1B.) Feel how your shoulders have softened and relaxed. Feel how your elbows have softened and now have a slight bend. Feel how your hands and fingers have softened. Feel how you can stretch lightly through the shoulders, arms, and hands without strain.

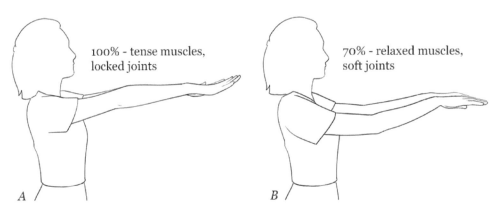

*Figure 3-1: The 70% Rule.*

Because your upper back, shoulders, arms, wrists, hands, and fingers have relaxed, circulation of blood and other fluids in these areas has increased. This contributes to the overall health of the tissues. If there were an injury in the area, that injury would receive more healing substances carried by blood and other fluids. That's a big point of the 70% Rule.

In summary, the 70% Rule directs us to:

- Feel our bodies
- Move within a range of motion that promotes relaxation, not tension
- Maintain our practice volume at a level where we don't feel strain

Following the 70% Rule in Tai Chi for Balance will accelerate your progress and help you avoid discomfort.

## Rule #2: The Don't Cause Pain Rule

Rule #2 holds:

**In Tai Chi for Balance, we do *not* move in ways that cause pain.**

Rule #2 works like this: In performing the movements of Tai Chi for Balance, if *any* movement causes pain, we adjust the movement so that we can perform it pain-free. This concept seems straightforward and sensible. But, in practice, it often requires major change.

Why? Because those of us who have experienced chronic pain tend to "push through the pain." We live with it, at least until we can tolerate the pain no longer.

Most often, pain is a signal that tissue is irritated, injured, or diseased. An overarching objective in any Tai Chi practice, including Tai Chi for Balance, is achieving vibrant health. We don't achieve vibrant health by moving in ways that cause pain. Instead of ignoring pain and "pushing through it," we listen carefully to pain signals and adjust our movements to minimize those signals.

Figure 3-2 depicts an example of Rule #2. Say you're shifting your weight forward, and you experience pain in the front ankle toward the end of the movement. (Figure 3-2A.)

Following the Don't Cause Pain Rule, you could shorten your stance and reduce the amount of weight you shift forward, until you were moving within a pain-free range of motion, *however small that range of motion may be.* (Figure 3-2B.)

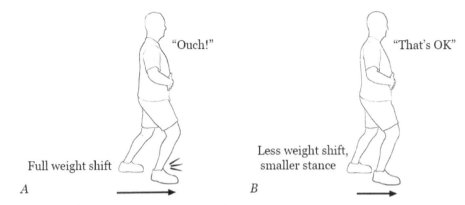

*Figure 3-2: The Don't Cause Pain Rule.*

In summary, the Don't Cause Pain Rule directs us to:

- Feel for pain
- Adjust our alignments and range of motion to eliminate pain

As you learn to perform Tai Chi for Balance movements without pain, the sensitivity and skill you develop will transfer to other parts of your life. You will soon find yourself making subtle adjustments in body alignments and range of motion in other activities in response to pain signals. Instead of "pushing through pain" and aggravating the underlying condition, you'll discover how to perform many activities in a pain-free manner.

With the Two Rules covered, let's proceed to the next chapter where we'll stand up and explore Neutral Posture.

## Chapter Wrap-Up

The Two Rules covered in this chapter apply to all we do in Tai Chi for Balance. Here's a quick recap.

- **Rule #1: The 70% Rule**: In Tai Chi for Balance, we perform all movements and all practices only up to 70% of our maximum.
- **Rule #2: The Don't Cause Pain Rule**: In Tai Chi for Balance, we do _not_ move in ways that cause pain. We adjust our movements until we can perform them pain-free.

By following the Two Rules, you'll accelerate your progress and maximize the potential for the Tai Chi for Balance System to support vibrant health.

# Chapter 4

# Neutral Posture, Feeling Your Feet, and Feeling Your Center

This chapter introduces three fundamental components of Tai Chi for Balance:

- ➢ Neutral Posture
- ➢ Feeling Your Feet
- ➢ Feeling Your Center

We incorporate these three components into exercises and movements throughout the program. Some, or all, of these may be new to you. That's okay. Just follow my guidance, and they'll soon become second nature.

## Neutral Posture

Tai Chi for Balance starts with a specific way to stand, a "posture." We call it **Neutral Posture**. One purpose of Neutral Posture is to organize the body into an upright, balanced, relaxed structure. We then can more clearly feel what's going on in our bodies.

In Tai Chi for Balance, Neutral Posture provides a platform for developing more **Whole Body Awareness**. In particular, Neutral Posture will help you **Feel Your Feet** and **Feel Your Center**. With practice, you'll develop increasingly consistent awareness of your feet and your center, helping you maintain a stable structure, a key to avoiding falls.

We build Neutral Posture from the ground up with 5 Basic Alignments. Some of the alignments may feel unusual at first. For most of us, it's a new way to position the body. With a little practice, you'll find your body settles into this posture comfortably and naturally

**The 70% Rule applies.** Before covering specifics, an important reminder. The 70% Rule applies here. If an alignment causes strain or discomfort, that's a signal that you have exceeded your 70% for that alignment. Just back off. Adjust the alignment until you are comfortable. With practice, tight spots in your body begin to stretch and open, and you'll maintain the prescribed alignment with comfort.

**The 5 Basic Alignments.** We build Neutral Posture from the ground up, establishing the following 5 Basic Alignments.

1. **Feet parallel, under the hips**. Start by positioning your feet parallel, approximately under the hips. (Figure 4-1.)

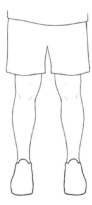

*Figure 4-1: Feet parallel, under the hips.*

With the feet parallel, under the hips, you'll feel your weight drop down your legs, into your feet, then into the floor.

2. **Knees unlocked**. Next, feel your knees. If your knees are locked, unlock them so there is a slight bend in the knees. (Figure 4-2.)

*Neutral Posture, Feeling Your Feet, Feeling Your Center*

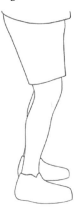

*Figure 4-2: Knees unlocked.*

With your knees unlocked, you'll get a feeling of softness in your knees. You'll know you've got it when you can gently bounce and feel your knee joints comfortably absorb the bounce, like shock absorbers.

3. **Tailbone relaxed down.** Next, feel your lower back and behind your pelvis. Then gently relax that area. When you do, your tailbone will rotate slightly forward and down. (Figure 4-3.) We'll call this "relaxing the tailbone down."

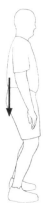

*Figure 4-3: Tailbone relaxed down.*

As you relax your tailbone down, you'll feel a gentle release and slight lengthening in the lower spine and behind the pelvis.

4. **Midriff open.** Next, feel your midriff. That's the area in the front of your abdomen between the top of your hips and the bottom of your ribcage. Gently lift and open

your midriff. With your midriff open, rather than collapsed, you feel more space in your midsection. (Figure 4-4.)

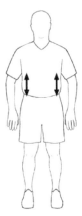

*Figure 4-4: Midriff open.*

To get a feel for this alignment, place your palms on either side of the front of your abdomen, between the bottom of the ribcage and the top of the hips. Then breathe deeply, using your breath to help open the area under your palms. When you exhale, maintain as much space there as you comfortably can.

5. **Occiput lifted.** We continue the gentle lifting from the midriff, up the spine to where the spine meets the skull, the occiput. To find your occiput, take a finger and feel behind your head where your spine meets your skull. Then gently lift the occiput, allowing your chin to rotate down. With your occiput lifted, you'll feel a light stretch in the back of the neck. (Figure 4-5.)

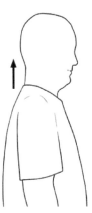

*Figure 4-5: Occiput lifted.*

*Neutral Posture, Feeling Your Feet, Feeling Your Center*

Computer and smartphone use have resulted in many people having a chronic head-forward, "tech neck" posture. This contributes to strain and discomfort in the shoulders, upper back, and neck. Lifting the occiput counteracts this. Over time, by lifting the occiput, you'll be able to comfortably move your head back over your neck, shoulders, and spine, helping you regain an upright, relaxed posture.

To review, the 5 Basic Alignments of Neutral Posture are:

1. Feet parallel, under the hips
2. Knees unlocked
3. Tailbone relaxed down
4. Midriff open
5. Occiput lifted

By establishing the 5 Basic Alignments of Neutral Posture, we organize our bodies into a more balanced, vertical, relaxed posture. (Figure 4-6.)

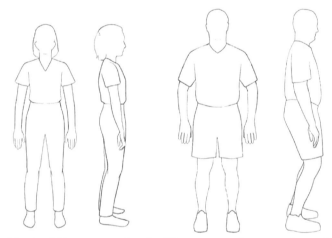

*Figure 4-6: Neutral Posture, 5 Basic Alignments, front and profile views.*

Once you get the 5 Basic Alignments together, you can add 3 Additional Adjustments, described in the next section.

TAI CHI FOR BALANCE

## The 3 Additional Adjustments

1. **Arms relaxed at the sides, a sense of openness in the armpits**. (Figure 4-7.)

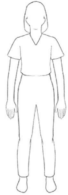

*Figure 4-7: Arms relaxed at sides, armpits open.*

This adjustment helps release the upper back, shoulders, and neck while improving circulation to and from the arms and hands. Allow your arms to hang from your shoulders, rather than holding the weight of your arms with your shoulder and back muscles. Rotate your arms so your palms face behind you. Let the thumb and index finger of each hand rest on the side of each thigh. Adjust your armpits so you have a light sense of openness in them.

2. **Relax the chest, open the back**. (Figure 4-8.)

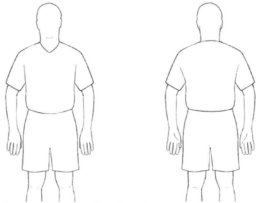

*Figure 4-8: Relax the chest, open the back.*

This adjustment continues releasing the back, neck, and shoulders while relaxing the chest. First, allow your back to expand, getting a sense of the shoulder blades moving slightly away from the spine. Then, relax your chest, getting a sense of your chest releasing and sinking. To be clear, this does *not* mean slumping forward, collapsing your posture. You maintain your 5 Basic Alignments while you relax the chest.

3. **Balance the pressure in your feet**. (Figure 4-9.)

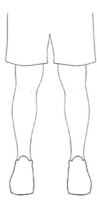

*Figure 4-9: Balance the pressure in your feet.*

Feel the pressure in your feet created by the force of your weight contacting the floor. With small adjustments of your posture, balance that pressure between your feet so that each foot supports the same amount of your weight. Then balance the pressure on each foot so that the pressure is roughly even between the ball, the heel, and the sides of each foot.

To review, the 3 Additional Adjustments are:

1. Arms relaxed at the sides, a sense of openness in the armpits.
2. Relax the chest, open the back.
3. Balance the pressures in your feet.

With the 5 Basic Alignments and 3 Additional Adjustments, you will have established a balanced, centered, vertical structure. Plus, you will have begun the process of releasing tension without collapsing your posture.

**Using Neutral Posture**

Neutral Posture provides a stable, balanced structure for the body and a foundation for developing Whole Body Awareness. From Neutral Posture, you'll discover how to feel your feet and your center with increasing clarity and consistency, an important step toward maintaining a stable, falls-resistant structure.

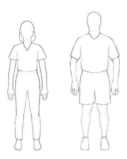

In Tai Chi for Balance, you'll begin and conclude each exercise in Neutral Posture.

# Feeling Your Feet

Developing Whole Body Awareness is the first of three main learning objectives in Tai Chi for Balance. You'll start by **feeling your feet**.

Human feet evolved to be sensitive, flexible, and mobile. Feet are rich with nerve endings, constantly transmitting signals to the brain. Those signals include pressure, position, and tactile sensations—like the qualities of the walking surface beneath us or contact with other objects. Those signals provide immensely helpful information for maintaining a stable structure and avoiding falls.

The problem is this: **Most people today do not feel their feet**. We bind them into footwear and bang around on them as we walk. This tends to decrease foot sensitivity.

Moreover, in our society, we tend to spend most of our time with "our minds in our heads." We pay almost constant attention to our thoughts, ignoring many of the physical sensations generated by the body's nerves. As a result, we rarely perceive the sensations transmitted from our feet.

If you've fallen, a version of this post-fall comment may sound familiar:

"I was walking along, and all of sudden I crashed to the ground."

If you've had this experience, at the moments leading up to your fall, you were not feeling your feet. Your mind was elsewhere, focused on thoughts unrelated to walking and avoiding a fall.

By ignoring our feet, we miss key sensations—like how a walking surface became slick from water, snow, or ice—increasing the risk of a slip. Or how our foot contacted a branch, rock, or other object that could trip us.

By developing sensitivity and skill at consistently feeling our feet, we can detect and respond to sensations that signal an increased risk of falling. In Tai Chi for Balance, you'll develop that sensitivity and skill.

With that, let's turn to our first Tai Chi for Balance exercise.

## Exercise 1: Feeling Your Feet

1. **Stand and settle into Neutral Posture**. Start by standing comfortably, settling into Neutral Posture. First, establish the 5 Basic Alignments described earlier. Then incorporate the 3 Additional Adjustments.

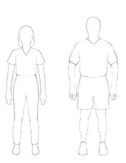

2. **Feel your body**. Then take a minute or so (or more if you want) and feel your body, starting at the top of your head and ending at your feet. This short practice helps you get your mind out of your head and into your body.

3. **Feel your feet**. Next, direct your awareness to your feet. Feel them. Small movements like wiggling your toes and gently rocking back and forth can help.

There's lots to feel. Your toes. The balls of your feet. Your heels. Your arches. Allow some time to feel your hard-working feet!

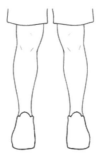

4. **Feel the pressure in your feet**. Next, focus your awareness on the sense of pressure in your feet. The sensation of pressure comes from the weight of your body contacting the floor through the soles of your feet. Feel how that pressure is distributed. Do you feel more pressure on the inside or outside of your feet? The balls of your feet? Your heels?

Next, let's start moving that pressure.

5. **Move some pressure to the balls of your feet**. With small movements of your legs, hips, and torso, move some pressure to the balls of your feet. (Figure 4-10.) Keep it light. Make small movements until you feel the pressure in your feet move slightly toward the front. Then pause and feel the sensation of having more pressure on the balls of your feet.

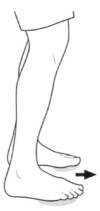

*Figure 4-10: Move a little pressure toward the balls of your feet.*

6. **Move some pressure to your heels**. Next, with small movements of your legs, hips, and torso, move some pressure to your heels. (Figure 4-11.) Pause and feel the sensation of having more pressure in your heels.

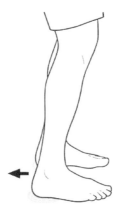

Figure 4-11: Move a little pressure toward your heels.

7. **Move some pressure to the right sides of your feet**. Next, move some pressure to the right side of each foot. (Figure 4-12.) Pause and feel the sensation of having more pressure on the right side of each foot.

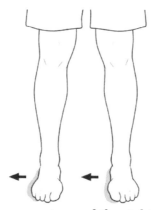

Figure 4-12: Move a little pressure toward the right sides of your feet.

8. **Move some pressure to the left sides of your feet**. Next, move some pressure to the left side of each foot. (Figure 4-13.) Pause and feel the sensation of having more pressure on the left side of each foot.

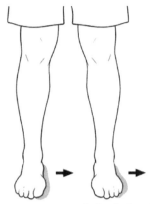

*Figure 4-13: Move a little pressure toward the left sides of your feet.*

9. **Continue to move the pressure in your feet to the balls, heels, right side, and left side.** Begin to gently move the pressure around your feet. For example, you can make circles with the pressure in the bottoms of your feet. (Figure 4-14.)

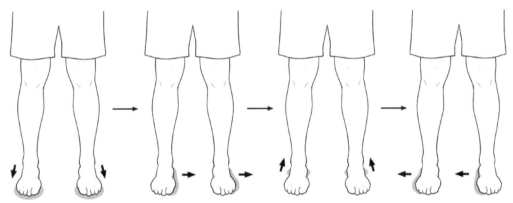

*Figure 4-14: Move the pressure around your feet.*

10. **Balance the pressure in your feet.** (Figure 4-15.) Next, balance the sensation of pressure between each foot and on each foot.

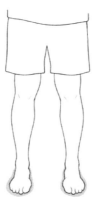

*Figure 4-15: Balance the pressures in your feet.*

11. **Conclusion**. Stand in Neutral Posture for a minute, or more if you like, continuing to feel your feet.

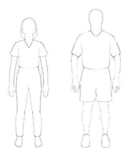

**Practice Recommendation:** Practice Exercise 1 for 2–4 minutes, take a break, then repeat. Do this for 2–3 sessions or more, as necessary, until you can clearly feel, and move, the pressure in your feet. Feel free to spread this practice over a day or more. When you've got that, you're ready for the next exercise. It's time to feel your center.

# Feeling Your Center

For starters, let me explain what I mean by "your center." In Tai Chi for Balance, I define your center as the line from the top of your head, your "Crown Point," straight down through the center of your body to the bottom of your pelvis, your perineum. (Figure 4-16.)

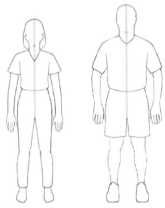

*Figure 4-16: Your center.*

Like most of the body, your center is rich with nerve endings. Those nerves constantly transmit information to the brain. One set of sensations transmitted from our center comes from our sense of **proprioception**, the sense of where the body or part of the body is in space. Proprioception helps us feel if our center is vertical or leaning.

Feeling your center provides a key to increasing stability and avoiding falls. As we explored in Chapter 2, when your posture is vertical, you're more stable. When you lean, you're less stable.

Without training and practice, most people don't feel their center. It's deep inside. Our awareness tends to be superficial and external. Or we're not feeling our body at all, focusing instead on the thoughts in our heads.

In Tai Chi for Balance, you'll soon develop a clear sense of your center. Even more important, you'll develop a clear sense of when your center is vertical and when it's not.

With that, let's turn to Exercise 2, and begin to feel our center.

# Exercise 2: **Feeling Your Center**

1. **Stand and settle into Neutral Posture.** Start by standing comfortably, settling into Neutral Posture. First, establish the 5 Basic Alignments described earlier. Next, incorporate the 3 Additional Adjustments.

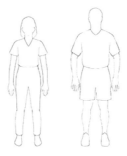

2. **Feel your body.** Then take a minute or so (or more if you want) and feel your body, starting at the top of your head and ending at your feet. This short practice helps you get your mind out of your head and into your body.

3. **Feel your Crown Point.** Next, direct your awareness to the top of your head, your Crown Point. (Figure 4-17.) Let your awareness stabilize there for a minute or so, feeling whatever you feel. Your hair, skin, the top of your skull. There's lots to feel.

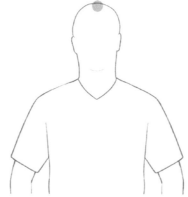

*Figure 4-17: Feel your Crown Point.*

4. **Feel straight down from your Crown Point.** Next, gradually drop your awareness straight down from your Crown Point. Through the center of your head.

Through the center of your neck. Through the center of your chest. Through the center of your abdomen. Take as much time as you want. There's lots to feel along the way. (Figure 4- 18A.) Continue dropping your awareness straight down until you arrive at the bottom of your pelvis, your perineum. (Figure 4- 18B.)

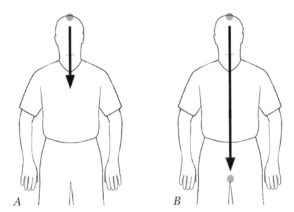

Figure 4-18: Feeling your center.

5. **Feel your center.** After taking a tour from your Crown Point to your perineum, feel for any sense of a line between those two parts of you. That's your center. Let your awareness stabilize there for a minute or two or more if you like. (Figure 4-19.)

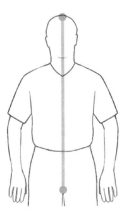

Figure 4-19: Feel your center.

6. **Position your center in the vertical.** Next, position your center so it's vertical. That is, not leaning. Checking visually in a mirror can help. It's common for people to think they are standing "straight," when they're leaning in one direction or

## Neutral Posture, Feeling Your Feet, Feeling Your Center

another, often leaning slightly back. When you position your center vertically as best as you can, take a moment to feel what that feels like. (Figure 4-20.)

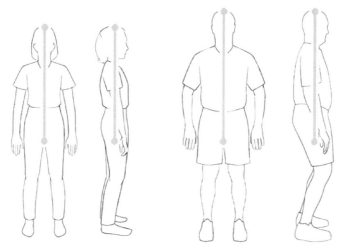

Figure 4-20: Position your center in the vertical.

7. **Lean your center slightly forward.** Now it's time to move your center. Lean your center slightly forward, just a few degrees off the vertical. (Figure 4-21.) Stabilize there for a moment and feel your center.

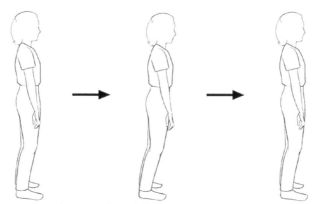

Figure 4-21: Leaning forward and feeling your center.

8. **Return your center to the vertical.** Feel how that feels. It feels different than when you're leaning forward.

9. **Lean your center slightly back.** Next, lean your center slightly back, just a few degrees off the vertical. (Figure 4-22.) Stabilize there for a moment. Feel your center leaning back.

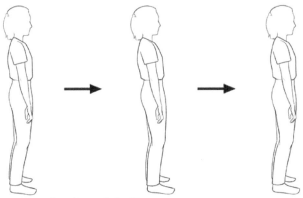

*Figure 4-22: Leaning back and feeling your center.*

10. **Return your center to the vertical.** Feel how that feels.

11. **Lean your center slightly to the right.** Next, lean your center slightly to your right side, just a few degrees off the vertical. (Figure 4-23.) Stabilize there for a moment. Feel your center leaning slightly right.

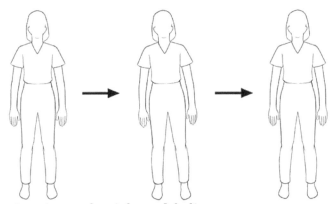

*Figure 4-23: Leaning to the right and feeling your center.*

12. **Return your center to the vertical.** Feel how that feels.

13. **Lean your center slightly to the left.** Next, lean your center slightly to the left, just a few degrees off the vertical. (Figure 4-24.) Stabilize there for a moment. Feel your center leaning slightly left.

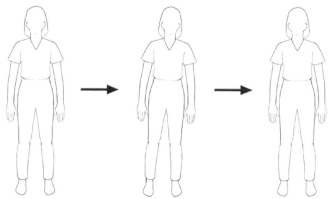

*Figure 4-24: Leaning to the left and feeling your center.*

14. **Return your center to the vertical.** Feel how that feels.

15. **Continue to lean your center and return it to the vertical**. For another 2-3 minutes, continue to slightly lean your center in one direction or another. Pause and feel. Then move your center back to the vertical. Pause and feel. (Figure 4-25) Repeat several times, leaning slightly in different directions.

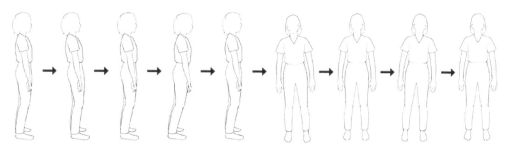

*Figure 4-25: Move your center around and back to the vertical.*

16. **Conclusion**. Move your center back to the vertical. Stand in Neutral Posture for a minute and notice how you feel after focusing your attention on feeling your center.

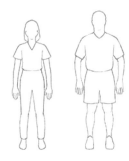

**Practice Recommendation**: Practice Exercise 2 for 3–4 minutes, take a break, then repeat. Do this for 2–3 sessions or more, as necessary, until you can feel your center and can clearly feel the difference between when your center is vertical and when it is leaning. When you've got that, you're ready for the next exercise. It's time to feel your feet *and* center.

## Exercise 3: Feeling Your Feet and Center

1. **Stand and settle into Neutral Posture**. Start by standing comfortably, settling into Neutral Posture. First, establish the 5 Basic Alignments described earlier. Next, incorporate the 3 Additional Adjustments.

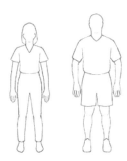

2. **Feel your feet**. Direct your awareness to your feet. Give yourself some time and feel what you can feel.

*Neutral Posture, Feeling Your Feet, Feeling Your Center*

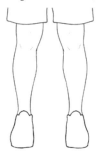

3. **Balance the pressure in your feet.** Next, adjust the position of your legs, hips, and torso as needed to balance the pressure between each foot and on each foot.

4. **Feel your feet and center.** Maintaining awareness of your feet, extend your awareness to the top of your head, your Crown Point. From there, drop your awareness straight down the center of your body to your perineum. Feel for the sense of a line between those two parts of you. Feeling as much of that line as you can, let your awareness stabilize there for a minute or two.

5. **Position your center in the vertical.** If your center is not already vertical, position it in the vertical. At the same time feel your feet. (Figure 4-26.) How does aligning your center vertically affect the sensation of pressure in your feet?

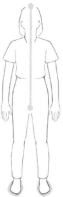

*Figure 4-26: Feeling your feet and center.*

6. **Lean your center slightly forward.** Next, lean your center slightly forward, just a few degrees off the vertical. (Figure 4-27.) Stabilize there for a moment, feeling your feet and center. Feel how leaning your center forward affects the sensation of pressure in your feet.

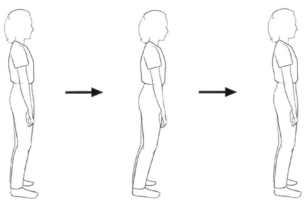
*Figure 4-27: Lean slightly forward, feeling your feet and center.*

7. **Return your center to the vertical.** Feel your feet. What changed?

8. **Lean your center slightly back.** Next, lean your center slightly back, just a few degrees off the vertical. (Figure 4-28.) Stabilize there for a moment, feeling your feet and center. Feel your feet. What happened?

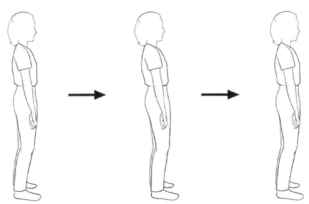
*Figure 4-28: Lean slightly back, feeling your feet and center.*

9. **Return your center to the vertical.** Feel how that affects the sensation of pressure in your feet.

10. **Lean your center slightly to the right.** Next, lean your center slightly to your right, just a few degrees off the vertical. (Figure 4-29B.) Stabilize there for a moment. Feel your feet. What happened?

*Neutral Posture, Feeling Your Feet, Feeling Your Center*

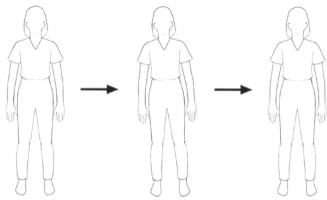

*Figure 4-29: Lean slightly to the right, feeling your feet and center.*

11. **Return your center to the vertical.** Feel how that affects the sensation of pressure in your feet.

12. **Lean your center slightly to the left.** Next, lean your center slightly to your right, just a few degrees off the vertical. Stabilize there for a moment, feeling your feet and center. (Figure 4-30.) What changed in your feet?

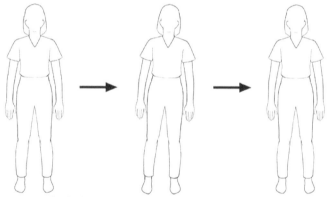

*Figure 4-30: Lean slightly to the left, feeling your feet and center.*

13. **Return your center to the vertical.** Feel how that affects the sensation of pressure in your feet.

14. **Continue to lean your center and return it to the vertical while feeling your feet and center**. For another 2-3 minutes, continue to lean your center a little in one direction or another. Pause and feel your feet and center. Then move

your center back to the vertical. Pause and feel. (Figure 4-31) Repeat several times, leaning slightly in different directions.

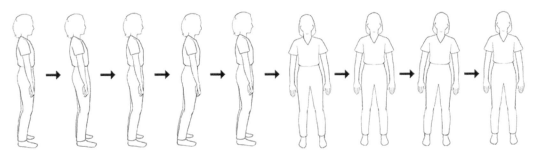

*Figure 4-31: Continue to lean your center and return to the vertical.*

15. **Conclusion**. Stand in Neutral Posture for a minute and notice how you feel after focusing your attention on feeling your feet and center.

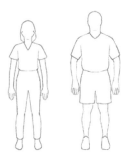

Here are the main takeaways from this exercise:

- By feeling your feet, you can discern sensations that help you maintain a more vertical posture.
- By feeling your center, you can discern sensations that help you balance the pressure in your feet.

In this way, feeling your feet and center reinforce each other in helping you maintain a more stable structure.

**Practice Recommendation:** Practice Exercise 3 for 3–4 minutes, take a break, then repeat. Do this for 2–3 sessions or more, until you can maintain your awareness of

*Neutral Posture, Feeling Your Feet, Feeling Your Center*

your feet <u>and</u> your center. In doing so, you'll develop increasing sensitivity in feeling when you're unintentionally leaning. From that awareness, you'll increase your skill in adjusting your posture back to the vertical—all while gathering important information from your feet.

Feel free to spread this practice over a day or more. When you've got that, you're ready to move. For that, turn to Part 2.

# Chapter Wrap-up

This chapter covered fundamental components of the Tai Chi for Balance System. Here's a recap of key points.

**Neutral Posture**

Neutral Posture provides an upright, balanced, vertical structure, helping us feel the body in detail and release tension. Neutral Posture includes **the 5 Basic Alignments**:

1. Feet parallel, under the hips
2. Knees unlocked
3. Tailbone relaxed down
4. Midriff open
5. Occiput lifted

After establishing the 5 Basic Alignments, we add **3 Additional Adjustments**:

1. Arms relaxed at the sides, a sense of openness in the armpits
2. Relax the chest, open the back
3. Balance the pressures in your feet

**Feeling Your Feet**

In Tai Chi for Balance, one key sensation is the feeling of pressure in your feet. You can feel when the pressure is balanced on each foot. You can feel when that pressure is more toward the ball, heel, or the sides of a foot.

**Feeling Your Center**

We define our center as the line between the top of the head, or Crown Point, straight down to the bottom of the pelvis, the perineum. By feeling your center, you can feel when your posture is vertical. You can feel when you are leaning. By feeling your center, you can more consistently maintain a vertical posture.

**Feeling Your Feet and Your Center**

By extending your awareness to both your feet and your center, you feel how changes in your posture change the pressure in your feet. These sensations provide additional information to help you maintain a more stable structure.

# Part 2

# Beginning to Move:

# Vertical Circles

In Part 2, we build upon the previous exercises, assembling the first movements of our Tai Chi for Balance Exercise Set. "Assembling movements" describes the teaching approach I use to help people efficiently learn and benefit from Tai Chi movements.

It goes like this: We start by learning the separate components of an exercise. For example, we first learn the movements of the legs and the hips. Then we learn the movements of the arms and hands. Next, we combine those components, coordinating multiple "moving parts." Then we refine the combined components into an increasingly smooth, connected, whole-body movement.

Once you get a feel for the basic movement, you'll progress to performing the movement while feeling your feet and center.

Then we repeat that process with the next exercise.

The lower-body movement components introduced in Part 2 include the Kwa Squat, the Weight Shift, the Hip Turn + Kwa Fold, and the Weight Shift + Hip Turn. The upper-body movements involve circling the arms and hands in the vertical plane (also called the "sagittal plane"). We will call these movements "Vertical Circles."

Separated into nine chapters, Part 2 contains the most material of this book's five parts. I encourage you to take your time with Part 2. With a little practice, you'll soon perform the movements with increasing coordination, confidence, and enjoyment. Most of the material in Part 2 is incorporated into the movements presented in Parts

3 and 4. By taking the time to get clear on the material in Part 2, you will find Parts 3 and 4 straightforward.

Before proceeding, a short Practice Note with an overview of the exercise set we're about to explore—Tai Chi Circling Hands.

---

**Practice Note: Overview of Tai Chi Circling Hands®**

Developed by my main teacher, Master Bruce Frantzis, Tai Chi Circling Hands provides a Tai Chi-based movement set that is easy to learn and enjoyable to practice. Tai Chi Circling Hands consists of the following seven movements:

Circle #1: Vertical Circles + Kwa Squat
Circle #2: Vertical Circles + Weight Shift
Circle #3: Vertical Circles + Weight Shift + Hip Turn
Circle #4: Horizontal Circles + Kwa Squat
Circle #5: Horizontal Circles + Weight Shift + Hip Turn
Circle #6: Coronal Circles + Kwa Squat
Circle #7: Coronal Circles + Weight Shift + Hip Turn

Performing a full set of Circling Hands involves repeating each of the seven movements 20 times, with direction changes and stance changes. A full set takes about 15-20 minutes, providing a low impact, yet thorough, whole-body workout.

In Tai Chi for Balance, as you learn and practice Tai Chi Circling Hands, your Whole Body Awareness will grow, as will your skill at maintaining Precise Posture Control. Along the way, your legs and hips will gain strength and flexibility. With that, you'll develop a more stable, fall-resistant structure.

Many aspects of Tai Chi Circling Hands—including related Qigong practices, therapeutic applications, and other benefits—are beyond the scope of this book. For more information about Tai Chi Circling Hands, plus an excellent online course led by Master Frantzis, go to https://www.energyarts.com/tai-chi-for-beginners/.

---

Let's proceed to Chapter 5 and start to move.

# Chapter 5

## Connecting the Bottom to the Top: The Kwa Squat

Tai Chi involves connected, whole-body movement. A collection of Chinese writings known as the "Tai Chi Classics" contains an artful description of this characteristic of Tai Chi (translations vary):

*In Tai Chi:*

*When one part moves, all parts move.*
*When one part stops, all parts stop.*

Connected, whole-body movement helps give Tai Chi the smoothness, fluidity, and coordination you see from the outside. On the inside, connected, whole-body movement contributes to Tai Chi's ability to exercise the body deeply and generate impressive force.

For starters, to achieve connected, whole-body movement, we need to connect the bottom half of the body (feet, legs, hips, and pelvis) to the top half of the body (torso, shoulders, arms, neck, and head). In Tai Chi for Balance, we connect the bottom and top halves of the body by moving through a part of the body the Chinese call the "*kwa*."

The *kwa* roughly corresponds to the inguinal fold, the diagonal "bikini cut" lines on the front of the hip. The *kwa* includes that area on the surface of the body and deeper into the pelvis on both sides. I will refer to the *kwa* often in this book, and it will help you to get familiar with this area of your body. The next exercise provides a quick procedure for finding and feeling your *kwa*.

# Exercise 4: Finding Your *Kwa*

1. **Stand and settle into Neutral Posture.**

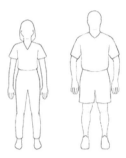

2. **Find the top of the sides of your hip bones.** With your fingers, find the tops of your hip bones on either side. Press in lightly and feel bone. (Figure 5-1A.)

3. **Find the top of the front of your hip bones.** With your index and middle fingers, walk around the tops of your hip bones to the front until your fingers are roughly aligned below your nipples. Press in lightly and feel bone. (Figure 5-1B.)

4. **Find the front of your kwa.** From there, walk your fingers straight down, 2–3 inches, until you reach a "squishy spot" of soft tissue. When you get it, you've found the center of the front of your kwa on both sides. (Figure 5-1C.)

5. **Feel your kwa.** Let your mind settle into the area beneath your fingers.

6. **Repeat.** Repeat steps 2–5 until you can readily find and feel your *kwa*.

## Connecting the Bottom to the Top: The Kwa Squat

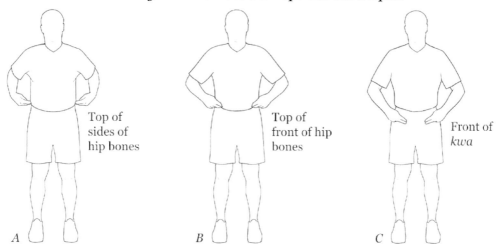

Figure 5-1: Finding your kwa.

In the Tai Chi for Balance System, you'll learn to move your *kwa* in two distinct ways. If *kwa*-centered movement feels unusual at first, don't worry. Just follow my guidance, and you'll soon get the hang of it.

The **Kwa Squat** is a key component in our movement set. You'll perform the Kwa Squat in 3 of the 7 movements of Tai Chi Circling Hands. The elements of a Kwa Squat are straightforward. Coordinating those elements takes most of us some practice. To introduce the Kwa Squat, I'll start with the Basic Elements.

## Basic Elements

1. **Stand and settle into Neutral Posture**. Then place your hands lightly on your abdomen. (Figure 5-2A)

2. **Sink into a Kwa Squat**. In one movement, allow your pelvis to sink down and back as you incline your torso forward, hinging at the *kwa*. (Figure 5-2B.) The amount of forward movement of the torso is proportional to the amount of downward and backward movement of the pelvis. Keep your knees stable over your feet.

3. **Rise back into Neutral Posture**. (Figure 5-2C.) In one movement, move your pelvis up and forward, as you move your torso back to vertical. Keep your knees stable over your feet.

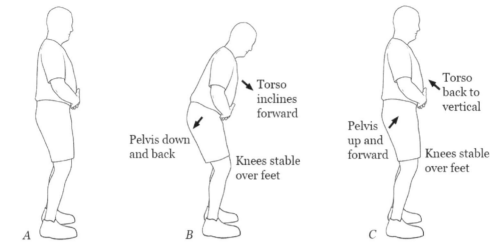

Figure 5-2: *The Kwa Squat.*

As you begin to practice the Kwa Squat, I recommend you reference the *Tips and Common Errors* in the next section. Following the tips and correcting the common errors helps most people perform an accurate beginning Kwa Squat in short order.

## Tips and Common Errors

*Tips*

**Maintain basic alignments.** Throughout the movement, maintain the Neutral Posture alignments of tailbone relaxed down, midriff open, and occiput lifted. In doing so, you move the torso, neck, and head as a unit.

**Keep the movements small.** At first, the Kwa Squat presents a coordination challenge for most of us. It's easier to coordinate when you keep the movements small. For example, you may want to start moving your pelvis down and back just 1–2 inches while inclining your torso a few degrees forward. As your coordination stabilizes, you can experiment with larger ranges of motion.

**Keep the movements relaxed.** The Kwa Squat does **not** involve squeezing, thrusting, or strong contractions. The abdomen, back, hips, and legs **remain relaxed**. For example, to initiate the squat, let gravity help pull your pelvis back and down as you incline your torso forward. Then, lightly press your feet into the floor and stretch up through your legs and kwa to bring your pelvis up and forward as you move your torso back to vertical.

**Feel your *kwa*.** As you perform the movements, extend your awareness into your *kwa*. Placing your index and middle fingers lightly in the center of your *kwa* on each side can help. Remember: The *kwa* is the hinge for the movement. As the coordination comes together, you will feel a gentle compression or "squish" in the *kwa* during the squat and a light stretch through the *kwa* as you come out of the squat.

**Common Errors**

**Torso inclines, pelvis does not move.** The backward movement of the pelvis and the forward inclination of the torso are coordinated and proportional. A common error is leaning the torso forward with little or no movement of the pelvis. (Figure 5-3A.)

**Flexing the spine instead of hinging at the *kwa*.** As the pelvis moves backward, the torso inclines forward, hinging at the *kwa*. A common error is flexing the spine, curling the torso, neck, and head forward. (Figure 5-3B.)

**Knees moving forward or back, not stable over the feet.** Throughout the Kwa Squat, the knees remain stable over the feet, not moving forward or back. For most, this is tricky at first. We are not used to stabilizing our knees this way. Common errors involve the knees moving forward during the squat or moving back while rising out of the squat. (Figure 5-3C.)

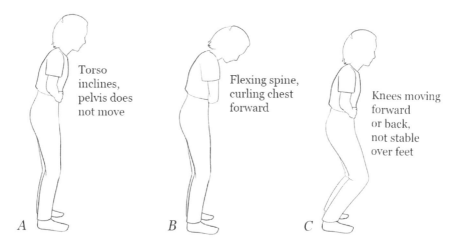

*Figure 5-3: The Kwa Squat, common errors.*

With that, let's proceed to Exercise 5.

## Exercise 5: The Kwa Squat

1. **Getting Ready to Move.** Stand and settle into Neutral Posture. Take a minute, or more if you like, and stand quietly before moving.

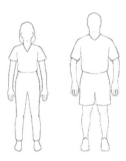

2. **Starting Position.** Place your hands lightly on your abdomen. (Figure 5-4A.)

3. **Sink into a Kwa Squat.** Allow your pelvis to sink down and back as you incline your torso proportionally forward. Keep your knees soft and stable over your feet. (Figure 5-4B.)

4. **Rise out of the Kwa Squat, back to Neutral Posture.** Bring your pelvis forward and up as your torso returns to the vertical. (Figure 5-4C).

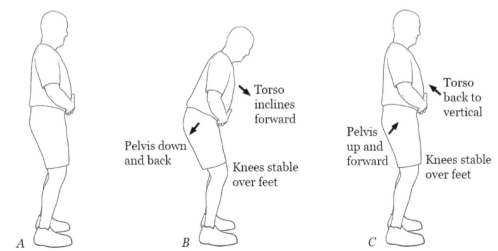

*Figure 5-4: The Kwa Squat.*

5. **Repeat**. Perform 20 repetitions.

6. **Conclusion**. Smoothly return to Neutral Posture.

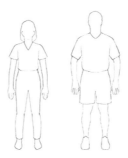

**Practice Recommendation:** For the first two weeks of Tai Chi for Balance, I recommend you do Exercise 5 daily, 1–3 times each day. It only takes a few minutes and will help to stabilize the coordination of the Kwa Squat. As you add other exercises, Exercise 5 serves as a good warm-up.

When you feel comfortable performing 20 Kwa Squats, you're ready for the next exercise. It's time to add feeling your feet and center.

# Exercise 6: Kwa Squat + Feeling Your Feet and Center

For the movements of Exercise 6, you can reference the instructions and figures for Exercise 5.

1. **Getting Ready to Move.** Take a minute, or more if you like, and stand quietly before moving. First, settle into Neutral Posture. Then feel your feet, balancing the pressure in your feet. Then feel your center, aligning your center vertically. Place your hands lightly on your abdomen.

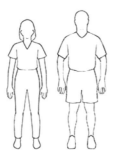 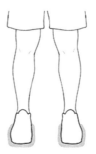 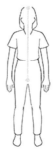

2. **Perform 20 Kwa Squats**. As you move, feel your feet and center. After each Kwa Squat, balance the pressure in your feet. After each Kwa Squat, return your center to the vertical.

3. **Conclusion**. Smoothly return to Neutral Posture.

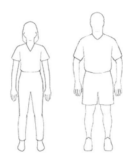

**Practice Recommendation:** Perform Exercise 6 for 1–2 days, 2–3 times per day. When you can perform 20 Kwa Squats while consistently feeling your feet and center, you're ready for the next chapter.

## Chapter Wrap-Up

This chapter introduced the Kwa Squat. You'll perform Kwa Squats in 3 of the 7 movements of the Tai Chi Circling Hands. Key points include:

**Kwa Squat**

To sink into a Kwa Squat:

- Allow your pelvis to sink down and back.
- Incline your torso forward, hinging at the *kwa*.
- The movement of your torso is proportional to the movement of your pelvis.
- Keep your knees stable over your feet.

To rise out of the Kwa Squat:

- Move your pelvis up and forward.
- Move your torso back to the vertical.
- Keep your knees stable over your feet.

As you perform the Kwa Squat, the goal is to remain relaxed, moving slowly and smoothly. This will help you develop increasingly connected, coordinated, whole body movement.

**Developing Whole Body Awareness**

- Performing Kwa Squats may change the pressure in your feet. You're aiming to become increasingly aware of that pressure and how it changes.
- Performing Kwa Squats involves aligning your center in the vertical, inclining your center forward, then returning it to the vertical. You're aiming to become increasingly aware when you center is vertical and when it's not.

# Chapter 6

## Adding the Arms: Vertical Circles

Tai Chi's movements are predominately circular, incorporating arcs, circles, spheres, and spirals. This circular nature of Tai Chi movements helps to deeply work virtually all the tissues of the body, with many health benefits validated by Western medical research.

For more information on the powerful health benefits of Tai Chi, I recommend the books *Tai Chi: Health for Life* by Bruce Frantzis (https://www.energyarts.com/books-by-bruce-frantzis/) and *The Harvard Medical School Guide to Tai Chi* by Peter Wayne, PhD.

To explore circular movement, we'll begin with the first type of circle in our movement set—the **Vertical Circle**. For starters, the Vertical Circle has four reference points:

- Back of the Vertical Circle
- Top of the Vertical Circle
- Front of the Vertical Circle
- Bottom of the Vertical Circle

As you arc your hands through these reference points, your hands will make Vertical Circles. To familiarize yourself with Vertical Circles, start with the Basic Elements below.

## Basic Elements

1. **Starting position, Back of Vertical Circle**. Place your hands in front you, roughly at the height of the bottom of your rib cage, about a fist's distance away from your skin, palms facing each other. This is the Back of your Vertical Circle. (Figure 6-1.)

# TAI CHI FOR BALANCE

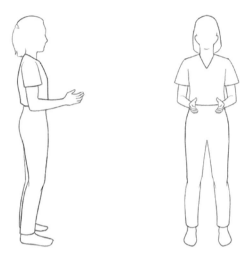

Figure 6-1: Back of Vertical Circle, profile and front views.

2. **Top of Vertical Circle**. Raise and extend your arms until your hands are positioned at about the level of your chin and several inches away from your body. This is the Top of your Vertical Circle. (Figure 6-2A.)

3. **Front of Vertical Circle**. Continue to extend your arms and hands in front of you, lowering them to approximately the level of your heart. Keep your elbows unlocked and shoulders soft. This is the Front of your Vertical Circle. (Figure 6-2B.)

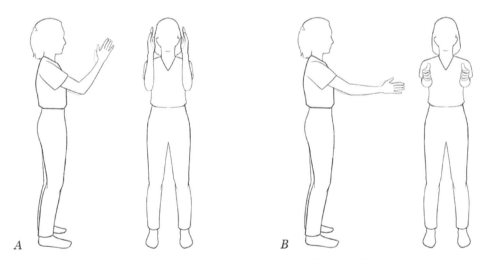

Figure 6-2: Top and Front of Vertical Circle, profile and front views.

*Adding the Arms: Vertical Circles*

4. **Bottom of your Vertical Circle**. Bend your arms and lower them to approximately the level of your hips, moving your hands back roughly halfway toward your body. This is the Bottom of your Vertical Circle. (Figure 6-3A).

5. **Back of your Vertical Circle**. Continue to bend and raise your arms, returning your hands to the Back of your Vertical Circle. (Figure 6-3B.)

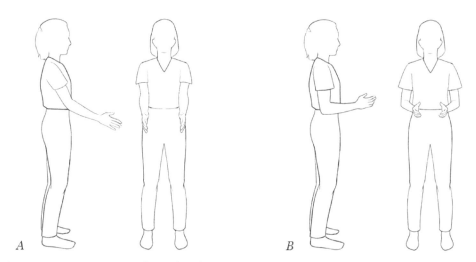

*Figure 6-3: Bottom and Back of Vertical Circle, profile and front views.*

6. **Make Top to Bottom Vertical Circles**. From the Back of your Vertical Circle, move your arms and hands through the positions again: Top, Front, Bottom, and Back of your Vertical Circle. Figure 6-4 shows those movements in sequence. I'll refer to circles in this direction as "Top to Bottom Vertical Circles." (Figure 6-4.)

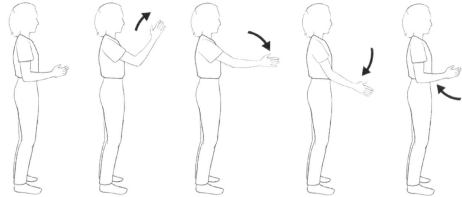

*Figure 6-4: Top to Bottom Vertical Circles.*

7. **Change directions; make Bottom to Top Vertical Circles**. From the Back of your Vertical Circle, change the direction of your circle, moving your arms and hands through the reference points as follows: Bottom, Front, Top, and Back of your Vertical Circle. Figure 6-5 shows those movements in sequence. I'll refer to circles in this direction as "Bottom to Top Vertical Circles."

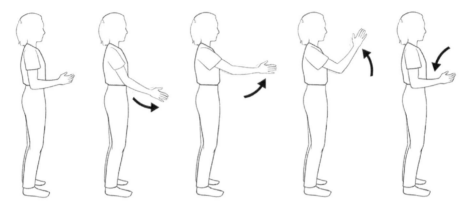

*Figure 6-5: Bottom to Top Vertical Circles.*

As you begin to practice Vertical Circles, I recommend you reference the *Tips and Common Errors* in the next section. Following the tips and correcting the common errors will help you perform smooth, circular Vertical Circles in short order.

## Tips and Common Errors

### *Tips*

**Keep the movements small.** Initially, many people find making smooth, circular Vertical Circles trickier than expected. Keeping your Vertical Circle smaller can help, say the size of a basketball rather than a beach ball. Once that stabilizes, you can experiment with different size circles, including large, medium, and small circles.

**Keep the movements relaxed.** The Vertical Circle does **not** involve tensing the shoulders, arms, hands, or any other body part. By releasing tension and relaxing, you will find it easier to move in a smooth, circular manner.

**Feel the stretch and release in your upper back, shoulders, and neck.** As you perform the movements, feel your upper back, shoulders, and neck. As the arms

## Adding the Arms: Vertical Circles

circle forward, you'll feel a light stretch. As the arms circle back, you'll feel the stretch release. With practice, the sensations of stretch and release become smooth and continuous.

### *Common Errors*

**Not making circles.** A circle is a constant distance around a central point. A common error is to make a non-circular shape with the arms and hands. For example, an oval or a shape with flat spots in back or on top. Distortions in your Vertical Circle often reflect tightness and tension in the shoulders, upper back, and neck. (Figure 6-6A).

**Lifting the shoulders at the top of the circle.** Through all our movements, we want to keep the shoulders relaxed and soft. A common error is lifting the shoulders toward the Top of the Vertical Circle. This induces unnecessary tension. (Figure 6-6B).

**Locking the elbows at the front of the circle.** The 70% Rule applies to all our movements, including Vertical Circles. A common error when moving the hands toward the Front of the Vertical Circle is to stretch toward 100% and lock the elbows. This induces unnecessary tension. (Figure 6-6C).

**Leaning forward at the front of the circle.** We aim to maintain a vertical center, except when intentionally inclining it. A common error is leaning forward as we extend our arms forward. This results in a less stable structure. (Figure 6-6D).

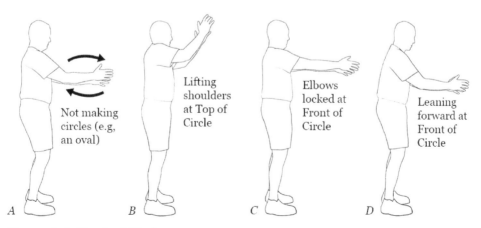

*Figure 6-6: Vertical Circles, common errors.*

# TAI CHI FOR BALANCE

With those Basic Elements, tips, and commons errors as guidance, let's proceed to Exercise 7.

## Exercise 7: Vertical Circles

1. **Getting Ready to Move.** Stand and settle into Neutral Posture. Take a minute, or more if you like, and stand quietly before moving.

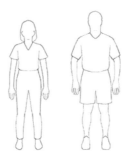

2. **Starting Position.** Position your hands at the Back of your Vertical Circle. (Figure 6-7A.)

3. **Make Top to Bottom Vertical Circles.** Begin circling your hands through the Top, Front, Bottom, and Back of your Vertical Circle. (Figure 6-7B-E.)

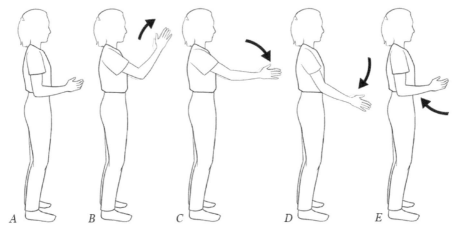

Figure 6-7: Top to Bottom Vertical Circles.

4. **Perform 10 repetitions.** After 10 repetitions, return to the Back of your Vertical Circle. (Figure 6-8A.)

*Adding the Arms: Vertical Circles*

5. **Change directions; make Bottom to Top Vertical Circles**. Change directions, circling through the Bottom, Front, Top, and Back of your Vertical Circle. (Figure 6-8B-E.)

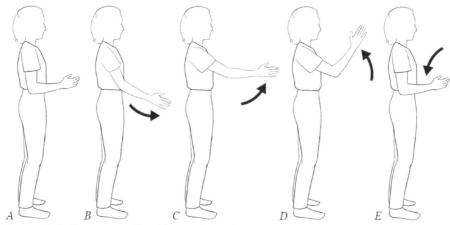

Figure 6-8: Bottom to Top Vertical Circles.

6. **Perform 10 repetitions**. After 10 repetitions, return to the Back of your Vertical Circle.

7. **Conclusion**. Smoothly transition to Neutral Posture.

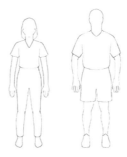

**Practice Recommendation.** Practice Exercise 6 for 1–2 days, 2–4 times per day. When you can comfortably make a set of 20 Vertical Circles, you're ready for the next exercise. It's time to add feeling your feet and center to your Vertical Circles.

# Exercise 8: Vertical Circles + Feeling Your Feet and Center

For the movements of Exercise 8, you can reference the instructions and figures for Exercise 7.

1. **Getting Ready to Move.** Take a minute, or more if you like, and stand quietly before moving. First, settle into Neutral Posture. Then feel your feet, balancing the pressure in your feet. Then feel your center, aligning it vertically.

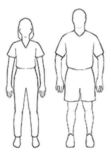 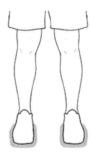 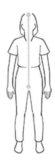

2. **Make Top to Bottom Vertical Circles, 10 repetitions.** As you move, feel your feet and center. Aim to maintain balanced pressures in your feet. Small pressure changes are okay. Aim to maintain your center in the vertical. After 10 repetitions, return to the Back of your Vertical Circle.

3. **Change directions, make Bottom to Top Vertical Circles, 10 repetitions.** As you move, maintain awareness of your feet and center as described above. After 10 repetitions, return to the Back of your Vertical Circle.

4. **Conclusion.** Smoothly transition to Neutral Posture.

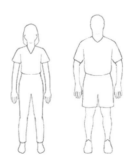

*Adding the Arms: Vertical Circles*

**Practice Recommendation:** You may find that making Vertical Circles while feeling your feet and center is easier said than done. Not to worry. Most of us have spent much of our life **not** feeling our feet or center. So, it's new. With a little practice, you'll soon develop the sensitivity to maintain increasingly constant awareness of your feet and center.

Practice Exercise 8 for 1–2 days, 2–3 times each day. When you can comfortably make a set of 20 Vertical Circles while feeling your feet and maintaining your center in the vertical, you're ready for the next chapter.

# Chapter Wrap-up

In this chapter, we began to explore circular movement, a key characteristic of Tai Chi. We start with Vertical Circles. Key takeaways include:

**Making Vertical Circles**

- Vertical Circles have four reference points, the Back, Top, Front, and Bottom.
- Ideally, each reference point is the same distance from the center point of the circle. As we arc our hands through those reference points, we make Vertical Circles.
- We extend the arms and stretch to circle the hands to the Front of the Vertical Circle. We bend the arms to circle the hands to the Back of the Vertical Circle.

**Vertical Circles–2 Directions**

- For Top to Bottom Vertical Circles, start at the Back of the Vertical Circle, then circle your hands through the Top, Front, Bottom, and Back of the Vertical Circle.
- For Bottom to Top Vertical Circles, start at the Back of the Vertical Circle, then circle your hands through the Bottom, Front, Top, and Back of the Vertical Circle.

**Developing   Whole Body Awareness and Precise Posture Control**

- Performing Vertical Circles will result in different patterns of pressure in your feet compared to Neutral Posture.
- Maintaining, or correcting to, balanced pressure in your feet while making Vertical Circles will help develop your foot sensitivity and awareness.
- Performing Vertical Circles may move your center off the vertical.
- Maintaining, or correcting to, a vertical center will help develop your postural awareness and control.

# Chapter 7

# Circle #1: Vertical Circles + Kwa Squat

In this chapter, we incorporate the material from Chapters 3–6 into Vertical Circles + Kwa Squat. Let's start with the Basic Elements.

## Basic Elements

1. **Starting Position**. Sink into a Kwa Squat. Position your hands at the Back of your Vertical Circle. (Figure 7-1.) We begin with Top to Bottom Vertical Circles.

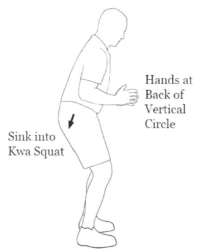

*Figure 7-1: Vertical Circles + Kwa Squat, Starting Position.*

2. **Top of Vertical Circle + Kwa Squat**. From the Starting Position, begin to rise from your Kwa Squat, as you extend your arms slightly and circle your hands to the Top of your Vertical Circle. (Figure 7-2A.)

3. **Front of Vertical Circle + Kwa Squat.** Complete rising out of the Kwa Squat until your torso is vertical, as you extend your arms and circle your hands to the Front of your Vertical Circle. (Figure 7-2B.)

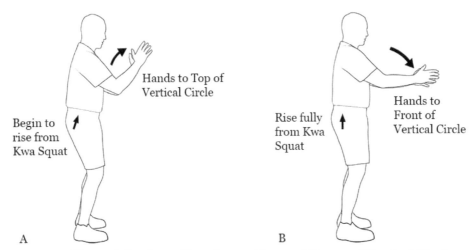

Figure 7-2: Vertical Circles + Kwa Squat, Top and Front of Vertical Circle.

4. **Bottom of Vertical Circle + Kwa Squat.** Begin to sink back into your Kwa Squat, as you bend your arms slightly, and circle your hands to the Bottom of your Vertical Circle. (Figure 7-3A.)

5. **Back of Vertical Circle + Kwa Squat.** Continue sinking into a Kwa Squat, as you bend your arms and circle your hands to the Back of your Vertical Circle. (Figure 7-3B.)

*Circle #1: Vertical Circles + Kwa Squat*

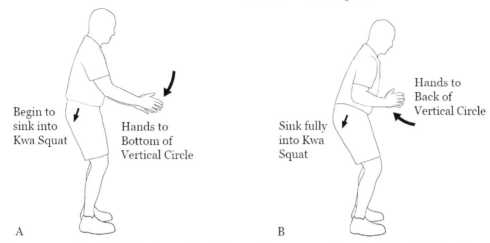

*Figure 7-3: Vertical Circles + Kwa Squat, Bottom and Back of Vertical Circle.*

Figure 7-4 shows the movements in sequence.

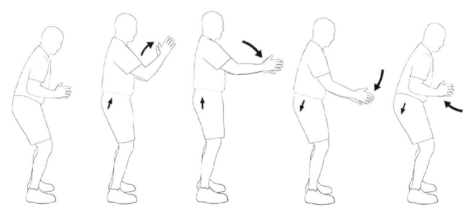

*Figure 7-4: Top to Bottom Vertical Circles + Kwa Squat.*

6. **Change directions**. Make Bottom to Top Vertical Circles + Kwa Squat.

7. **Bottom of Vertical Circle + Kwa Squat.** From the Back of your Vertical Circle, begin to rise from the Kwa Squat, as you extend your arms and circle your hands to the Bottom of your Vertical Circle. (Figure 7-5A.)

8. **Front of Vertical Circle + Kwa Squat.** Continue rising from your Kwa Squat until your torso is vertical, as you continue to extend your arms and circle your hands to the Front of your Vertical Circle. (Figure 7-5B.)

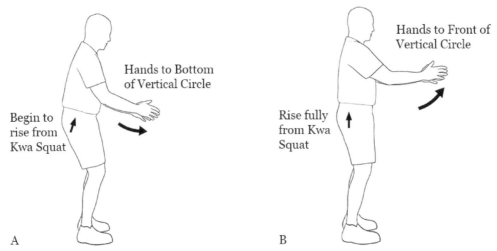

*Figure 7-5: Vertical Circles + Kwa Squat, Bottom and Front of Vertical Circle.*

9. **Top of Vertical Circle + Kwa Squat.** Begin to sink into a Kwa Squat, as you bend your arms slightly and circle your hands to the Top of your Vertical Circle. (Figure 7-6A.)

10. **Back of Vertical Circle + Kwa Squat.** Continue sinking into a Kwa Squat, as you bend your arms and circle your hands to the Back of your Vertical Circle. (Figure 7-6B.)

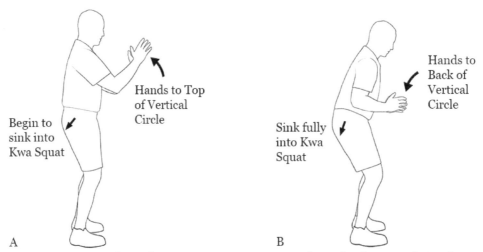

*Figure 7-6: Vertical Circles + Kwa Squat, Top and Back of Vertical Circle.*

Figure 7-7 shows the movements in sequence.

*Circle #1: Vertical Circles + Kwa Squat*

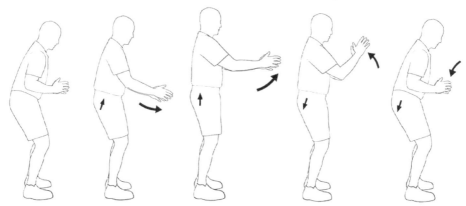

*Figure 7-7: Bottom to Top Vertical Circles + Kwa Squat.*

As you explore Circle #1, I encourage you to reference the *Tips and Common Errors* in the next section. Following the tips and correcting the common errors will help you rapidly perform Circle #1 in a smooth, connected manner.

## Tips and Common Errors

### *Tips*

**Connect your legs and waist to your arms and hands.** In Tai Chi, the legs and the waist power and control the arms and hands. Here, the "waist" refers to the *kwa*, the pelvis, the hip joints, the lower abdomen, and related muscles and soft tissue. In Circle #1, the Kwa Squat is the key to making this connection.

As you sink into the Kwa Squat, feel for a sense of the Kwa Squat drawing your arms and hands toward the Back of your Vertical Circle. As you rise out of the Kwa Squat, feel for a sense of the stretching of the legs and *kwa* powering your arms and hands toward the Front of your Vertical Circle.

**Feel for a sense of coordinated bending and stretching.** You'll find it helpful to get a sense of coordinated bending and stretching as you perform Circle #1. At the Back of your Vertical Circle, you are in a Kwa Squat, bending your hips, knees, and ankles. You're also bending your arms at the shoulder and elbow joints. You can also lightly bend your wrists, hands, and fingers.

At the Front of your Vertical Circle, you have come out of your Kwa Squat and can feel a light stretch through your legs and *kwa*. Your arms and hands have circled forward, and you can feel a light stretch through the arms, shoulders, and upper back. You can also lightly stretch your wrists, hands, and fingers. This sense of coordinated bending and stretching will help guide your movements.

## Common Errors

**Legs and arms out of phase.** A common error is for the legs and arms to get "out of phase." This happens when the legs stretch (rising out of the Kwa Squat) while the arms bend (moving toward the Back of the Vertical Circle). (Figure 7-8A.) It also happens when the legs bend (sinking into the Kwa Squat) while the arms stretch (moving toward the Front of the Vertical Circle). (Figure 7-8B.)

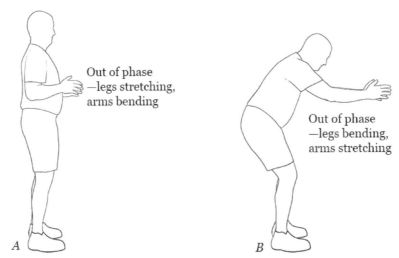

*Figure 7-8: Vertical Circle + Kwa Squat, common errors.*

With those Basic Elements, tips, and common errors in mind, let's turn to Exercise 9.

*Circle #1: Vertical Circles + Kwa Squat*

# Exercise 9: Vertical Circles + Kwa Squat

1. **Getting Ready to Move.** Stand and settle into Neutral Posture. Take a minute, or more if you like, and stand quietly before moving.

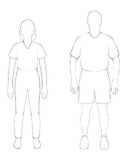

2. **Starting Position.** Sink into a Kwa Squat. Position your hands at the Back of your Vertical Circle. (Figure 7-9A.)

3. **Make Top to Bottom Vertical Circles, 10 repetitions.** From the Starting Position, rise from the Kwa Squat as you extend your arms and circle your hands through the Top and Front of your Vertical Circle. (Figure 7-9B-C.) Then sink into a Kwa Squat as you bend your arms and circle your hands through the Bottom and Back of your Vertical Circle. (Figure 7-9D-E). After 10 repetitions, return to the Back of your Vertical Circle.

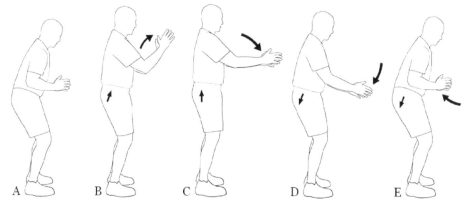

*Figure 7-9: Top to Bottom Vertical Circles + Kwa Squat.*

4. **Change directions; Make Bottom to Top Vertical Circles, 10 repetitions.** From the Back of your Vertical Circle, rise from the Kwa Squat as you extend your

arms and circle your hands through the Bottom and Front of your Vertical Circle. (Figure 7-10A-C.) Then sink into a Kwa Squat as you bend your arms and circle your hands through the Top and Back of your Vertical Circle. (Figure 7-10D-E). After 10 repetitions, return to the Back of your Vertical Circle.

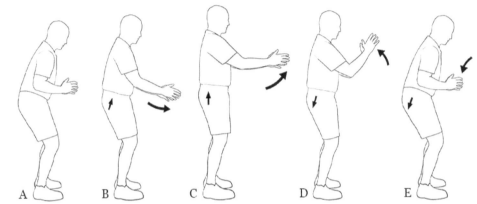

Figure 7-10: Bottom to Top Vertical Circles + Kwa Squat.

5. **Conclusion**. Smoothly transition to Neutral Posture.

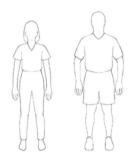

**Practice Recommendation:** Practice Exercise 9 for 1–3 days, 2–4 times per day. When you can comfortably make a set of 20 Vertical Circles + Kwa Squats, you're ready for the next exercise. It's time to add feeling your feet and center.

*Circle #1: Vertical Circles + Kwa Squat*

# Exercise 10: Vertical Circles + Kwa Squat + Feeling Your Feet and Center

For the movements of Exercise 10, you can reference the instructions and figures for Exercise 9.

**Practice Video.** You can also follow me in the guided practice video covering this exercise. To access the video, go to https://www.chicagotaichi.org/tai-chi-for-balance-guided-practice-videos/

1. **Getting Ready to Move.** Take a minute, or more if you like, and stand quietly before moving. First, settle into Neutral Posture. Then feel your feet, balancing the pressure in your feet. Then feel your center, aligning your center vertically.

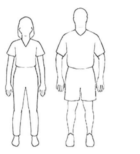 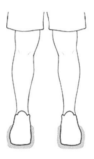 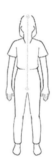

2. **Starting Position.** Sink into a Kwa Squat. Position your hands at the Back of your Vertical Circle.

3. **Make Top to Bottom Vertical Circles, 10 repetitions.** As you move, feel your feet and center. Before and after each Kwa Squat, balance the pressure in your feet and return your center to the vertical. After 10 repetitions, return to the Back of your Vertical Circle.

4. **Change directions; make Bottom to Top Vertical Circles, 10 repetitions.** As you move, feel your feet and center as described above. After 10 repetitions, return to the Back of your Vertical Circle.

5. **Conclusion.** Smoothly transition to Neutral Posture.

# TAI CHI FOR BALANCE

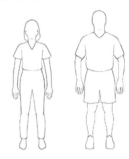

**Practice Recommendation:** Practice Exercise 10 for 1–3 days, 2–4 times per day. Note how your Whole Body Awareness and Precise Posture Control are developing. Can you more consistently keep track of your feet and your center as you move? With a little practice, you can do it!

When you can comfortably perform a set of 20 Vertical Circles + Kwa Squats while feeling your feet and center, you're ready for the next chapter.

# Chapter Wrap-up

This chapter introduced Vertical Circles + Kwa Squat, Circle #1 of our Tai Chi for Balance Exercise Set. Key points include:

**Make Vertical Circles by Coordinating the Kwa Squat and the Bending and Stretching of Your Arms**

- You want to develop a sense of making Vertical Circles mainly with the action of the legs and *kwa*, plus the bending and stretching of the arms.
- Sinking into the Kwa Squat plus bending the arms brings the hands to the Back of your Vertical Circle.
- Rising from Kwa Squat plus stretching the arms sends the hands to the Front of your Vertical Circle.

**Continuing to Develop Whole Body Awareness and Precise Posture Control**

- Performing Vertical Circles + Kwa Squat will result in different patterns of pressure in your feet compared to Neutral Posture.
- Maintaining, or correcting to, balanced pressure in your feet while making Vertical Circles + Kwa Squat will continue to develop your foot sensitivity and awareness.
- Performing Vertical Circles + Kwa Squat, while feeling your center and returning your center to the vertical after each repetition will continue to develop your postural awareness and control.

# Chapter 8

## Adding More Legs: The Weight Shift

A fundamental movement component of Tai Chi, and one source of its many health benefits, is the **Weight Shift**. We explore the Weight Shift in this chapter.

In Tai Chi, the Weight Shift involves the smooth, controlled, complete shifting of body weight from one leg to the other. In performing Tai Chi, you shift your weight in this manner almost constantly. For example, during a full set of Tai Chi for Circling Hands, you'll shift weight from one leg to the other *160 times*. That's exercise!

With regular practice, the Weight Shift in Tai Chi delivers the following benefits:

- Increases muscle strength in your hips and legs
- Increases tone of connective tissue in your hips and legs, including ligaments, tendons, and fascia
- Increases joint flexibility, especially in the feet and ankles
- Improves balance and stability
- Improves cardiovascular function
- May increase bone density in the lower extremities

Recall the #1 risk factor for falling in older adults—**loss of leg and hip strength**. The Weight Shift directly targets this risk factor. In short, there are lots of good reasons to incorporate the Weight Shift into your exercise regime.

At the same time, if you have issues with a foot, ankle, knee, hip, or your lower back, sometimes putting all your weight on one leg causes pain.

In Tai Chi for Balance, we aim to perform the Weight Shift pain-free. In this way, you will gain the health benefits of the Weight Shift, including stronger legs and hips, without aggravating existing conditions. The exercises in this chapter show you how.

> **Practice Note: Maximizing the Benefits of the Weight Shift**
>
> Three suggestions to help you maximize the benefits of the Weight Shift in Tai Chi for Balance:
>
> **Rule #1 applies: Stay within your 70%.** The Weight Shift requires muscular work and increases the forces on your muscles, joints, and connective tissues. Keep your range of motion and practice volume within a comfortable range.
>
> **Rule #2 applies: Don't cause pain.** Depending on what's going on in your body, a complete Weight Shift may cause discomfort. In that case, back off the size of the movement and the amount of weight shifted until your Weight Shift is pain-free. Initially, your Weight Shift may be much less than 100%. That's okay.
>
> **Slow down.** By moving more slowly, you'll find it easier to feel and adjust your alignments and movements to minimize discomfort.

Before exploring pain-free weight shifting, I'll introduce the Tai Chi for Balance Stance.

# The Tai Chi for Balance Stance

By "stance," I mean how we position our legs and feet when we perform exercises that include the Weight Shift, and later, the Weight Shift + Hip Turn. Our stance involves placing one foot forward with a small step and, if desired, rotating the back leg and foot out slightly. I will refer to our stances as **Left Leg Forward Stance** and **Right Leg Forward Stance**.

In this section, I describe the Tai Chi for Balance Stance and a way to change stances. First, I emphasize the two most important factors in establishing a stance in Tai Chi for Balance: *stability* and *comfort*. Put another way, when you put one foot forward, and start shifting weight, you want to feel stable, not wobbly. And you want your stance to feel comfortable, not causing strain or pain.

Establishing a stable, comfortable stance involves experimenting and making small adjustments. Typically, you'll adjust one or more of the following three variables:

- *Stance length* (how far you step forward)

## Adding More Legs: The Weight Shift

- *Stance width* (the lateral distance between your feet)
- *Back leg and foot position* (how much you rotate the back leg and foot out)

For example, if you step into a Left Foot Forward Stance, and you feel wobbly (Figure 8-1A), you may want to widen your stance, increasing the lateral distance between your feet. (Figure 8-1B.) As we covered in Chapter 2, you're widening your base of support to increase stability.

Similarly, if you feel too stretched out, making it difficult to shift weight (Figure 8-1C), then you may want to decrease your stance length, bringing your front foot closer to your back foot. (Figure 8-1D.)

If you feel strain in your back knee, ankle, or foot (Figure 8-1E), you may want to adjust your back leg and foot position, rotating a few degrees in or out. (Figure 8-1F.)

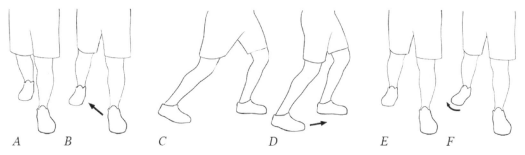

Figure 8-1: Adjusting your stance for stability and comfort.

How to adjust stance length, stance width, and back leg position for stability and comfort varies from person to person. When you take a stance, ask yourself, "Does this stance feel stable and comfortable?" If the answer is yes, great. Continue with the exercise. If the answer is no, then adjust your stance until you feel stable and comfortable.

One other point: The stability and comfort of a stance may change over the course of an exercise. A stance that feels fine at the start may benefit from adjustment later. If so, adjust it. During an exercise, when your weight is forward, you can adjust your back leg. When your weight is back, you can adjust your front leg.

With that, let's take a stance!

# The Tai Chi for Balance Stance

1. **Left Leg Forward Stance.** From Neutral Posture position, (Figure 8-1A) rotate your right leg and foot out slightly. Pivot on your right heel until your right leg and foot are rotated out 5-45 degrees. (Figure 8-2B.)

2. **Shift your weight to your right leg.** Shifting weight to the right leg prepares you to take a small step forward with your left leg. (Figure 8-2C.)

3. **Take a small step forward with your left leg.** To start, step so that your left heel lands 1"–3" beyond the toes of the right foot, with your heels remaining Neutral Posture distance apart. This is your Left Leg Forward Stance. (Figure 8-2D.)

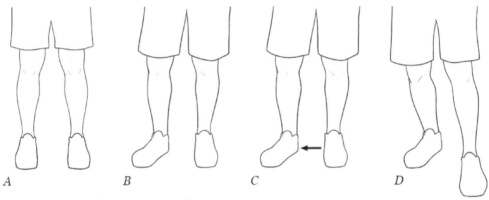

*Figure 8-2: Left Leg Forward Stance.*

4. **Adjust for stability and comfort.** Adjust your stance length, stance width, and rear leg and foot position until you feel stable and comfortable.

5. **Change to a Right Leg Forward Stance.** Now it's time to change stances. Shift weight to your back leg. Move your front leg and foot back to Neutral Posture position (Figure 8-3A.)

6. **Rotate your left leg and foot out slightly.** Pivot on your left heel until your left leg and foot are rotated out 5-45 degrees. (Figure 8-3B.)

7. **Shift your weight to your left leg.** Shifting weight to your left leg prepares you to take a small step forward with your right leg (Figure 8-3C.)

*Adding More Legs: The Weight Shift*

8. **Take a small step forward with your right leg.** Step so that your right heel lands 1"–3" in front of the toes of the left foot, with your heels remaining Neutral Posture distance apart. This is your Right Leg Forward Stance. (Figure 8-3D.)

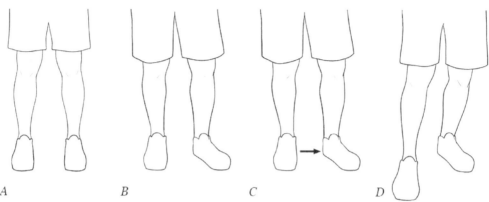

*Figure 8-3: Right Leg Forward Stance.*

9. **Adjust for stability and comfort.** Adjust your stance length, stance width, and rear leg and foot position until you feel stable and comfortable.

10. **Conclusion.** Shift weight to your back leg. Move your front leg and foot back to Neutral Posture position. Rotate your left foot back to Neutral Posture position.

I recognize those seem like detailed instructions for "put one foot forward, then put the other foot forward." I want us to have a baseline procedure for establishing and changing stances. You'll get ample practice in the exercises that follow. Soon, stepping into a stance, adjusting your stance for stability and comfort, and changing stances will become nearly automatic.

**A note about stance instructions in Tai Chi for Balance.** In all the exercises where we take a stance, I start with Left Leg Forward Stance, then change to Right Leg Forward Stance. This is for consistency only. If you prefer starting with Right Leg Forward Stance, go for it. When the instructions say change stances, then change to Left Leg Forward Stance.

With that, let's begin exploring the Weight Shift with Exercise 11.

# Exercise 11: The Weight Shift

1. **Getting Ready to Move.** Stand and settle into Neutral Posture. Take a minute, or more if you like, and stand quietly before moving.

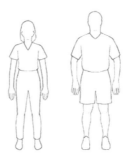

2. **Starting Position, Left Leg Forward Stance.** Adjust your stance length, stance width, and foot position for stability and comfort.

3. **Shift Weight.** Move your pelvis and torso back so that your weight is on your back leg. Bend your rear knee and hip so you feel like you are sitting on your back leg. (Figure 8-4A.) Then push with your back leg, shifting weight to your front leg. (Figure 8-4B.) Your front knee will bend, and your back knee and hip will extend. Then push with your front leg, shifting weight to your back leg. Your back leg and hip will bend, and your front knee and hip will extend. (Figure 8-4C.)

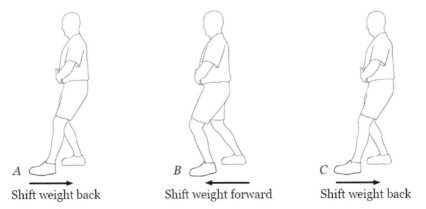

Figure 8-4: *The Weight Shift, left leg forward.*

4. **Perform 10 repetitions.** After 10 repetitions, shift weight back.

## Adding More Legs: The Weight Shift

5. **Change your stance to Right Leg Forward Stance.** Adjust your stance length, stance width, and foot position for stability and comfort.

6. **Shift Weight.** Shift weight back. Bend your rear knee and hip so you feel like you are sitting on your back leg. (Figure 8-5A.) Then push with your back leg, shifting weight to your front leg. (Figure 8-5B.) Your front knee will bend, and your back knee and hip will extend. Then push with your front leg, shifting weight to your back leg. Your back leg and hip will bend, and your front knee and hip will extend. (Figure 8-5C.)

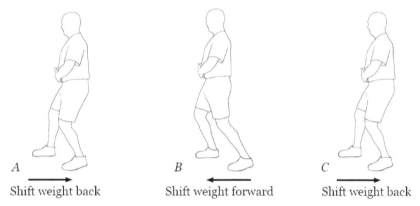

*Figure 8-5: The Weight Shift, right leg forward.*

7. **Perform 10 repetitions.** After 10 repetitions, shift weight back.

6. **Conclusion.** Smoothly transition to Neutral Posture.

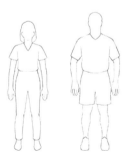

A simple exercise, I recognize. We shift weight all the time. For example, during normal walking, we completely shift weight during each step. Still, most people rarely, if ever, consciously focus on *how* they shift weight. Developing Whole Body Awareness and Precise Posture Control as we shift weight is a key to maintaining a more stable, fall-resistant structure.

**Practice Recommendation:** Practice Exercise 11 for 1–2 days, 2–4 times per day. When you can establish stable, comfortable stances, and shift weight from one leg to the other within a pain-free range of motion, you are almost ready for Exercise 12.

First, let's consider one common error when shifting weight.

## Common Error

**Leaning when shifting weight.** When shifting weight, most people lean in the direction of the weight shift. When shifting weight to the front leg, they lean forward. (Figure 8-6A.) When shifting weight to the back leg, they lean back. (Figure 8-6B.) As you know from Chapter 2, leaning results in a less stable structure. We want to eliminate leaning when shifting weight, **aiming to maintain a vertical posture**.

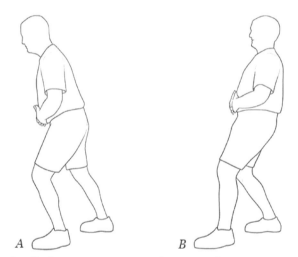

*Figure 8-6: Weight Shift common error, leaning the torso.*

With that, let's proceed to Exercise 12. Because of the common tendency to lean when shifting weight, we'll start by feeling our center as we shift weight.

*Adding More Legs: The Weight Shift*

# Exercise 12: Weight Shift + Feeling Your Center

1. **Getting Ready to Move.** Take a minute, or more if you like, and stand quietly before moving. First, settle into Neutral Posture. Then feel your center, aligning it vertically.

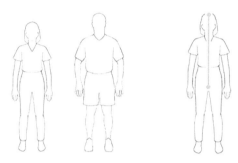

2. **Starting Position, Left Leg Forward Stance, weight back.** Adjust your stance for stability and comfort. Then shift weight back. Bend your rear knee and hip slightly so that you feel like you are sitting on your back leg. (Figure 8-7A.)

3. **Shift weight, maintaining a vertical posture**. Pushing with your back leg, shift weight forward. Pause. Feel your center. If you're leaning forward, align your center vertically. (Figure 8-7B.) Then pushing with your front leg, shift weight back. Pause. Feel your center. If you're leaning back, align your center vertically. (Figure 8-7C.)

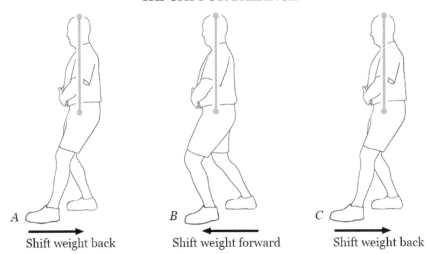

Figure 8-7: *The Weight Shift, left leg forward, maintaining vertical posture.*

4. **Perform 10 repetitions**. With each Weight Shift, check your center, and correct as needed.

5. **Change your stance to Right Leg Forward Stance.** Adjust your stance for stability and comfort. Shift weight back. (Figure 8-8A.)

6. **Shift weight, maintaining a vertical posture**. Pushing with your back leg, shift weight forward. (Figure 8-8B.) Then pushing with your front leg, shift weight back. (Figure 8-8C.) Align your center vertically as described above.

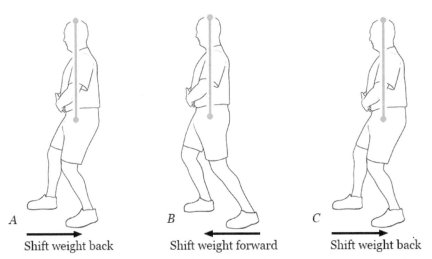

Figure 8-8: *The Weight Shift, right leg forward, maintaining vertical posture.*

*Adding More Legs: The Weight Shift*

7. **Perform 10 repetitions**. With each Weight Shift, check your center, and correct as needed.

8. **Conclusion**. Smoothly transition to Neutral Posture.

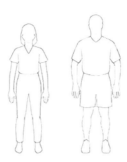

As you practice Exercise 11, you'll become increasingly aware of your posture as you shift weight. You'll gain proficiency at shifting weight while maintaining a more vertical posture.

**Practice Recommendation:** Practice Exercise 12 for 1–2 days, 2–4 times per day. When you have a clear sense of shifting weight while maintaining a vertical posture, you're ready for Exercise 13.

In Exercise 13, we incorporate feeling your feet into the Weight Shift. As we shift weight from one leg to the other, the pressure in our feet constantly changes, increasing in one foot, while decreasing in the other.

On each foot, you want to balance the pressure across the bottom of the foot, as the overall amount of pressure increases or decreases. Developing the sensitivity and skill to keep the pressure on a foot balanced as you shift weight is one key to developing Whole Body Awareness. In Exercise 13, you begin developing that sensitivity and skill.

TAI CHI FOR BALANCE

# Exercise 13: Weight Shift + Feeling Your Feet and Center

For the movements of Exercise 13, you can reference the instructions and figures for Exercise 12.

1. **Getting Ready to Move.** Take a minute, or more if you like, and stand quietly before moving. First, settle into Neutral Posture. Then feel your feet. Balance the pressure in your feet. Then feel your center. Align your center vertically.

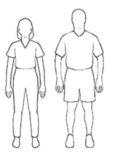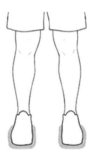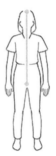

2. **Starting Position, Left Leg Forward Stance, weight back.** Adjust your stance for stability and comfort. Then shift weight back.

3. **Shift weight, 10 repetitions.** Pushing with your back leg, shift weight forward. Then, pushing with your front leg, shift weight back. As you move, feel your feet. Feel the pressure in your feet change as you shift weight. Feel your center. Maintain, or correct to, a vertical posture as you shift weight. After 10 repetitions, change your stance.

4. **Change to a Right Leg Forward Stance.** Adjust your stance for stability and comfort. Then shift weight back.

5. **Shift Weight, 10 repetitions.** As you move, feel your feet and center as described above. Maintain, or correct to, a vertical posture.

6. **Conclusion.** Smoothly transition to Neutral Posture.

*Adding More Legs: The Weight Shift*

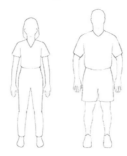

As you develop Whole Body Awareness while moving, you'll feel your feet and center with increasing consistency. You'll balance the pressure in each foot, even as those pressures constantly change. You'll maintain a more vertical posture with fewer corrections. Soon, you will perform Exercise 13 as smooth, continuous movement.

**Practice Recommendation:** Practice Exercise 13 for 1–2 days, 2–4 times per day. You can also use Exercise 13 as a warm-up before the exercises in the next chapter. When you have a clear sense of your ability to shift weight while feeling your feet and center, evenly distributing the pressure on each foot, and maintaining a vertical posture, you're ready for the next chapter.

# Chapter Wrap-up

This chapter covered another fundamental movement component of the Tai Chi for Balance System—the Weight Shift. Key points include:

**Left Leg Forward Stance and Right Leg Forward Stance**

- The stance involves placing one leg forward by taking a small step forward.
- The front foot is 1"-3" ahead of the toes of the back foot.
- The heels remain roughly Neutral Posture distance apart.
- You may rotate the back leg and foot out between 5-45 degrees.
- We adjust our stance for *stability* and *comfort*. Adjustments include stance length, stance width, and the angle of the back leg and foot.

**The Weight Shift**

- To shift weight forward, we push with the back leg.
- To shift weight back, we push with front leg.
- The weighted leg bends.
- The unweighted leg extends.
- As we shift weight, we maintain our center in the vertical.
- We perform the Weight Shift within a pain-free range of motion, adjusting the amount of the Weight Shift and our stance until the Weight Shift is pain-free.

**Honing Your Whole Body Awareness and Precise Posture Control**

- As we shift weight, the pressure on each foot constantly changes. We aim to feel those changes, and balance the pressure on each foot.
- As we shift weight, we aim to maintain a vertical posture. By feeling your center, you can detect and correct any tendency to lean as you move. This helps you develop increasingly Precise Posture Control.

# Chapter 9

## Circle #2: Vertical Circles + Weight Shift

In this chapter, you'll add Vertical Circles to your Weight Shift, forming Circle #2 Vertical Circles + Weight Shift.

As exercise, performing Vertical Circles + Weight Shift will:

- Exercise the legs and hips, strengthening and stretching muscles and connective tissue
- Work in and around the shoulder joints, stretching and releasing the shoulders, upper back, and neck, relieving chronic tension
- Train the nervous system to coordinate whole-body movement, using the Weight Shift to power and control your Vertical Circle

As part of the Tai Chi for Balance System, performing Vertical Circles + Weight Shift will continue to develop your Whole Body Awareness and Precise Posture Control. Circle #2 does all that while moving your body in a dynamic and functional way.

With that, let's proceed to Vertical Circles + Weight Shift, starting with the Basic Elements.

## Basic Elements

1. **Starting Position, Left Leg Forward Stance, weight back**. Adjust your stance for stability and comfort. Shift weight back. Place your hands at the Back of your Vertical Circle. (Figure 9-1.)

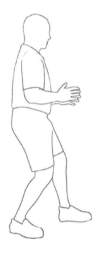

*Figure 9-1: Vertical Circles + Weight Shift, left leg forward, Starting Position.*

2. **Make Top to Bottom Vertical Circles + Weight Shift.** We'll start with Top to Bottom Vertical Circles + Weight Shift.

3. **Top of Vertical Circle.** From the Starting Position, push from your back leg, shifting half your weight to the front leg, as you extend and raise your arms and hands to the Top of your Vertical Circle. (Figure 9-2A.)

4. **Front of Vertical Circle.** Continue shifting weight forward, extending your arms and hands to the Front of your Vertical Circle. (Figure 9-2B.) Coordinate completing the Weight Shift forward with reaching the Front of the Vertical Circle.

*Circle #2: Vertical Circles + Weight Shift*

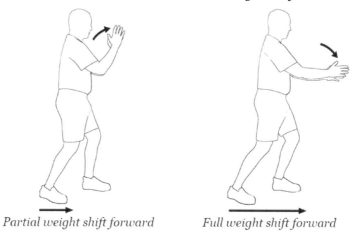

Partial weight shift forward         Full weight shift forward

*Figure 9-2: Vertical Circles + Weight Shift, left leg forward, Top and Front of Vertical Circle.*

5. **Bottom of Vertical Circle.** Pushing with the front leg, shift half your weight to the back leg, bending your arms and moving your hands to the Bottom of your Vertical Circle. (Figure 9-3A.)

6. **Back of Vertical Circle**. Continue shifting weight back, bending your arms and moving your hands to the Back of your Vertical Circle. (Figure 9-3B.) Coordinate completing the Weight Shift back with reaching the Back of the Vertical Circle.

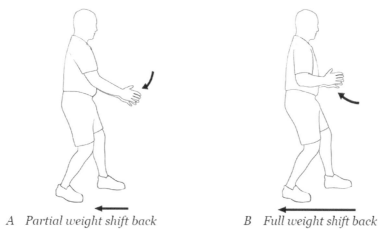

A   Partial weight shift back         B   Full weight shift back

*Figure 9-3: Vertical Circles + Weight Shift, left leg forward, Bottom and Back of Vertical Circle.*

Figure 9-4 shows those movements in sequence.

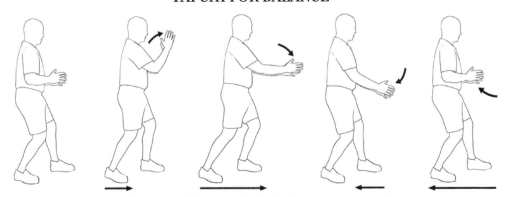

*Figure 9-4: Vertical Circles + Weight Shift, left leg forward, Top to Bottom Vertical Circles.*

7. **Change directions.** Make Bottom to Top Vertical Circles + Weight Shift.

8. **Bottom of Vertical Circle.** From the Back of your Vertical Circle, push from your back leg, shifting half your weight to the front leg as you extend your arms and hands to the Bottom of Vertical Circle. (Figure 9-5A.)

9. **Front of Vertical Circle.** Continue shifting weight forward, extending your arms and hands to the Front of your Vertical Circle. (Figure 9-5B.) Coordinate completing the Weight Shift forward with reaching the Front of the Vertical Circle.

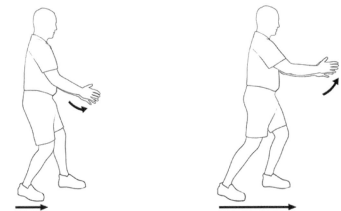

A  Partial weight shift forward     B  Full weight shift forward

*Figure 9-5: Vertical Circles + Weight Shift, left leg forward, Bottom and Front of Vertical Circle.*

*Circle #2: Vertical Circles + Weight Shift*

10. **Top of Vertical Circle.** Shift half your weight to the back leg as you bend your arms, moving your hands to the Top of your Vertical Circle. (Figure 9-6A.)

11. **Back of Vertical Circle.** Continue shifting weight back, bending your arms and moving your hands to the Back of your Vertical Circle. (Figure 9-6B.) Coordinate completing the Weight Shift back with reaching the Back of the Vertical Circle.

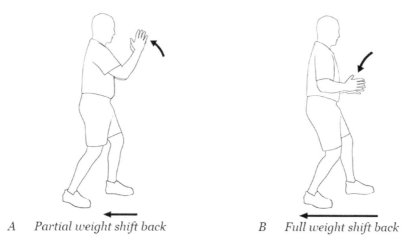

   A    Partial weight shift back        B    Full weight shift back

*Figure 9-6: Vertical Circles + Weight Shift, left leg forward, Top and Back of Vertical Circle.*

Figure 9-7 shows those movements in sequence.

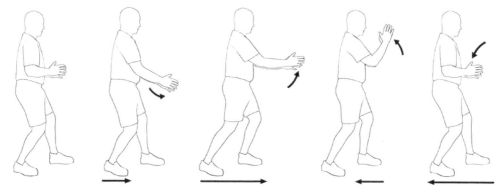

*Figure 9-7: Vertical Circles + Weight Shift, left leg forward, Bottom to Top Vertical Circles.*

12. **Change your stance, Right Leg Forward Stance, weight back.** Adjust your stance for stability and comfort. Shift weight back. Position your hands at the Back of your Vertical Circle. (Figure 9-8.) We'll start with Top to Bottom Vertical Circles.

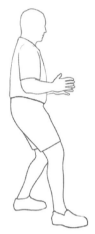

*Figure 9-8: Vertical Circles + Weight Shift, right leg forward, Back of Vertical Circle.*

13. **Top of Vertical Circle.** Push with your back leg, shifting half your weight to the front leg, as you extend your arms and hands to the Top of Vertical Circle. (Figure 9-9A.)

14. **Front of Vertical Circle.** Continue shifting weight forward, extending your arms and hands to the Front of your Vertical Circle. (Figure 9-9B.) Coordinate completing the Weight Shift forward with reaching the Front of the Vertical Circle.

### Circle #2: Vertical Circles + Weight Shift

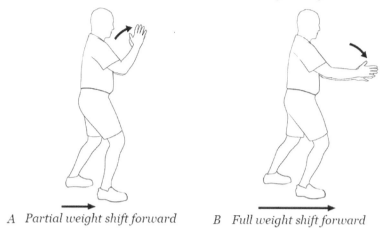

A  Partial weight shift forward    B  Full weight shift forward

*Figure 9-9: Vertical Circles + Weight Shift, right leg forward, Top and Front of Vertical Circle.*

15. **Bottom of the Vertical Circle.** Pushing with your front leg, shift half your weight to the back leg as you bend your arms and move your hands to the Bottom of your Vertical Circle. (Figure 9-10A.)

16. **Back of Vertical Circle.** Continue shifting weight back, bending your arms and moving your hands to the Back of your Vertical Circle. (Figure 9-10B.) Coordinate completing the Weight Shift back with reaching the Back of the Vertical Circle.

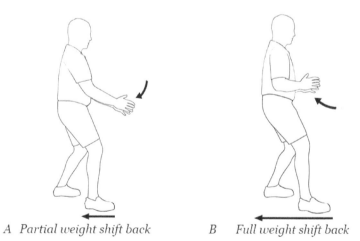

A  Partial weight shift back    B  Full weight shift back

*Figure 9-10: Vertical Circles + Weight Shift, right leg forward, Bottom and Back of Vertical Circle.*

Figure 9-11 shows those movements in sequence.

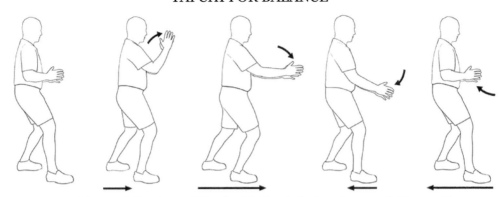

*Figure 9-11: Vertical Circles + Weight Shift, right leg forward, Top to Bottom Vertical Circles.*

17. **Change directions**. Make Bottom to Top Vertical Circles + Weight Shift.

18. **Bottom of Vertical Circle.** From the Back of your Vertical Circle, pushing with your back leg, shift half your weight to the front leg as you extend your arms and hands to the Bottom of the Vertical Circle. (Figure 9-12A.)

19. **Front of Vertical Circle.** Continue shifting weight forward, extending your arms and hands to the Front of your Vertical Circle. (Figure 9-12B.) Coordinate completing the Weight Shift forward with reaching the Front of the Vertical Circle.

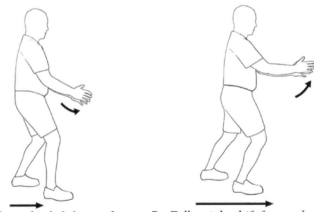

A   Partial weight shift forward    B   Full weight shift forward

*Figure 9-12: Vertical Circles + Weight Shift, right leg forward, Bottom and Front of Vertical Circle.*

## Circle #2: Vertical Circles + Weight Shift

20. **Top of the Vertical Circle.** Pushing with your front leg, shift half your weight to the back leg, as you bend your arms and move your hands to the Top of your Vertical Circle. (Figure 9-13A.)

21. **Back of Vertical Circle.** Continue shifting weight back, bending your arms and moving your hands to the Back of your Vertical Circle. (Figure 9-13B.) Coordinate completing the Weight Shift back with reaching the Back of the Vertical Circle.

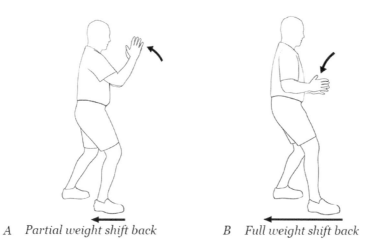

    A   *Partial weight shift back*           B   *Full weight shift back*

*Figure 9-13: Vertical Circles + Weight Shift, right leg forward, Top and Back of Vertical Circle.*

Figure 9-14 shows those movements in sequence.

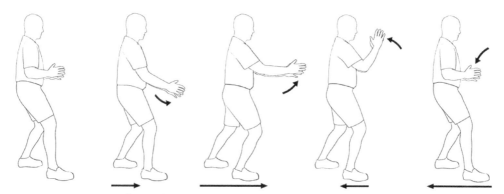

*Figure 9-14: Vertical Circles + Weight Shift, right leg forward, Bottom to Top Vertical Circles.*

As you begin to practice Vertical Circles + Weight Shift, I encourage you to reference the *Tips and Common Errors* in the next section. I also suggest you review the *Tips and Common Errors* sections in Chapter 6 (Vertical Circles) and Chapter 8 (Weight Shift).

By following the tips and correcting the common errors, plus a little practice, your Circle #2's will soon become increasingly smooth, connected, and enjoyable.

## Tips and Common Errors

### *Tips*

**The Weight Shift powers and controls your Vertical Circles.** As you perform Circle #2, relax and soften your shoulders. Let your elbows sink a little. Feel for any sense of your arms connecting to your back, rather than being lifted by your shoulder muscles.

As you shift weight forward, feel how the weight shift helps power your arms and hands toward the Front of your Vertical Circle. As you shift your weight back, feel how the weight shift helps draw your arms and hands toward the Back of your Vertical Circle.

**Balance the size of the Vertical Circle with the Weight Shift.** The ideal Weight Shift is 100% of your weight on one leg, then 100% of your weight on the other leg. That said, follow the 70% Rule and the Don't Cause Pain Rule, reducing the amount of the Weight Shift until you can move within a pain-free range of motion.

As you adjust your Weight Shift, correspondingly adjust the size of your Vertical Circle. If your Weight Shift is smaller, then make a smaller Vertical Circle. (Figure 9-15A-B.) As the size of your Weight Shift increases, increase the size of your Vertical Circle. (Figure 9-15C-D.) The key is a clear sense of balance between the movement of your legs and the movement of your arms.

## Circle #2: Vertical Circles + Weight Shift

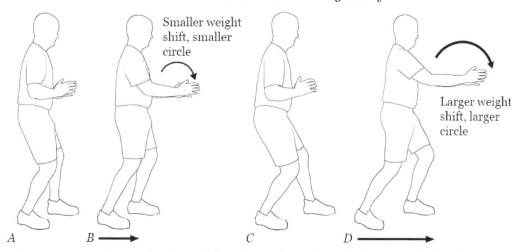

Figure 9-15: Balance the size of the Vertical Circle with the Weight Shift.

### Common Errors

**Leading with the arms and hands.** Tai Chi movement is powered by the legs and controlled by the waist. A common error is to lead the movements with the arms, reaching forward with the arms (Figure 9-16A), then pulling back with the arms. (Figure 9-16B.)

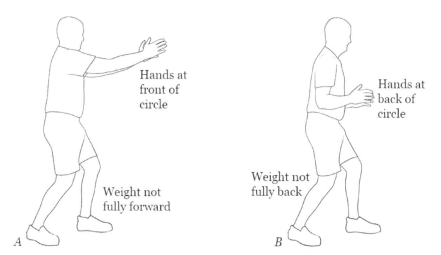

Figure 9-16: Vertical Circles + Weight Shift, common errors, leading with hands.

141

**Leaning.** We aim to maintain a vertical posture throughout the movement. A common error is to allow the arms to pull your torso forward or push the torso back, resulting in leaning. (Figure 9-17A-B).) This distorts your posture and results in a less stable structure.

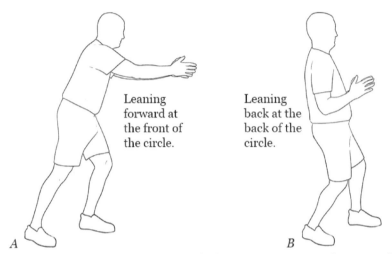

Figure 9-17: *Verticle Circles + Weight Shift, common errors, leaning the torso.*

With those Basic Elements, tips, and common errors in mind, let's proceed to Exercise 14.

## Exercise 14: Vertical Circles + Weight Shift

1. **Getting Ready to Move.** Stand and settle into Neutral Posture. Take a minute, or more if you like, and stand quietly before moving.

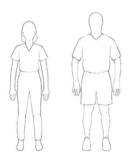

*Circle #2: Vertical Circles + Weight Shift*

2. **Starting Position, Left Leg Forward Stance, weight back**. Place your hands at the Back of your Vertical Circle. (Figure 9-18A.)

3. **Make Top to Bottom Vertical Circles, 5 repetitions**. From the Starting Position, smoothly shift weight forward as you extend your arms and hands through the Top and Front of your Vertical Circle. (Figure 9-18B-C.) Then smoothly shift weight back as you bend your arms and circle your hands through the Bottom and Back of your Vertical Circle. (Figure 9-18D-E.) After 5 repetitions, return to the back of your Vertical Circle.

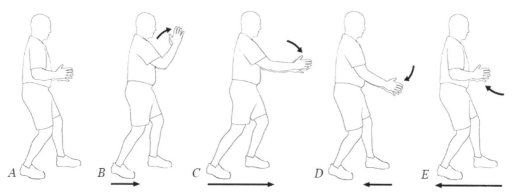

*Figure 9-18: Vertical Circles + Weight Shift, left leg forward, Top to Bottom Vertical Circles.*

4. **Change directions, make Bottom to Top Vertical Circles, 5 repetitions**. From the Back of your Vertical Circle (Figure 9-19A), smoothly shift weight forward as you extend your arms and hands through the Bottom and Front of your Vertical Circle. (Figure 9-19B-C.) Then smoothly shift weight back as you bend your arms and circle your hands through the Top and Back of your Vertical Circle. (Figure 9-19D-E.) After 5 repetitions, return to the Back of your Vertical Circle.

TAI CHI FOR BALANCE

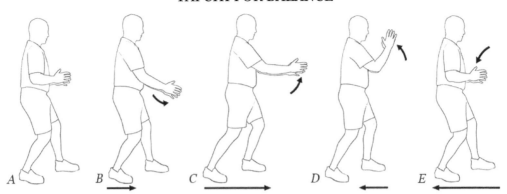

*Figure 9-19: Vertical Circles + Weight Shift, left leg forward, Bottom to Top Vertical Circles.*

5. **Change your stance to Right Leg Forward Stance**. Shift weight back. Place your hands at the Back of your Vertical Circle. (Figure 9-20A.)

6. **Make Top to Bottom Vertical Circles, 5 repetitions**. From the Back of Your Vertical Circle, smoothly shift weight forward as you extend your arms and hands through the Top and Front of your Vertical Circle. (Figure 9-20B-C.) Then smoothly shift weight back as you bend your arms and circle your hands through the Bottom and Back of your Vertical Circle. (Figure 9-20D-E.). After 5 repetitions, return to the Back of your Vertical Circle.

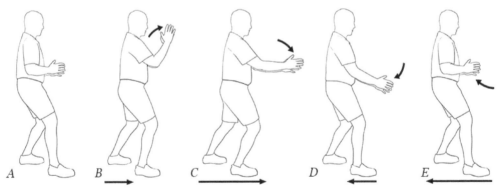

*Figure 9-20: Vertical Circles + Weight Shift, right leg forward, Top to Bottom Vertical Circles.*

7. **Change directions; make Bottom to Top Vertical Circles, 5 repetitions**. From the Back of your Vertical Circle (Figure 9-21A), smoothly shift weight forward, as you extend your arms and hands through the Bottom and Front of your

## Circle #2: Vertical Circles + Weight Shift

Vertical Circle. (Figure 9-21B-C.) Then smoothly shift weight back, as you bend your arms and circle your hands through the Top and Back of your Vertical Circle. (Figure 9-21D-E.) After 5 repetitions, return to the Back of your Vertical Circle

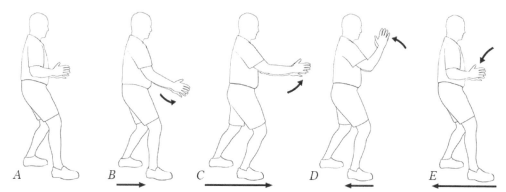

*Figure 9-21: Vertical Circles + Weight Shift, right leg forward, Bottom to Top Vertical Circles.*

8. **Conclusion**. Smoothly transition to Neutral Posture.

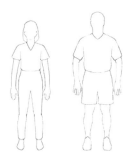

Following the Exercise 14 instructions, you'll complete 20 Vertical Circles + Weight Shifts, gradually increasing the volume of your Tai Chi for Balance exercises.

**Practice Recommendation:** Practice Exercise 14 for 1–2 days, 2–3 times per day. When you can comfortably make a set of 20 Vertical Circles with Weight Shifts, you're ready for the next exercise. It's time to add feeling your feet and center.

# Exercise 15: Vertical Circles + Weight Shift + Feeling Your Feet and Center

For the movements of Exercise 15, you can reference the instructions and figures for Exercise 14.

**Practice Video.** You can also follow me in the guided practice video covering this exercise. To access the video, go to https://www.chicagotaichi.org/tai-chi-for-balance-guided-practice-videos/

1. **Getting Ready to Move.** Take a minute, or more if you like, and stand quietly before moving. First, settle into Neutral Posture. Then feel your feet, balancing the pressure in your feet. Then feel your center, aligning your center vertically.

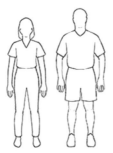 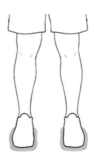 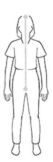

2. **Starting Position, Left Leg Forward Stance.** Shift weight back. Place your hands at the Back of your Vertical Circle.

3. **Make Top to Bottom Vertical Circles, 5 repetitions.** As you move, feel your feet. Feel the constantly changing pressure in each foot. Feel your center. Maintain, or correct to, a vertical posture. After 5 repetitions, return to the Back of your Vertical Circle.

4. **Change directions; make Bottom to Top Vertical Circles, 5 repetitions.** Feel your feet and center as described above. After 5 repetitions, return to the Back of your Vertical Circle.

5. **Change your stance to Right Leg Forward Stance.** Shift weight back.

*Circle #2: Vertical Circles + Weight Shift*

6. **Make Top to Bottom Vertical Circles, 5 repetitions.** Feel your feet and center as described above. After 5 repetitions, return to the Back of your Vertical Circle.

7. **Change directions; make Bottom to Top Vertical Circles, 5 repetitions.** Feel your feet and center as described above. After 5 repetitions, return to the Back of your Vertical Circle.

8. **Conclusion.** Smoothly transition to Neutral Posture.

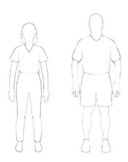

**Practice Recommendation:** Practice Exercise 15 for 1–3 days, 2–3 times each day. When you can comfortably make a set of 20 Vertical Circles + Weight Shifts while feeling your feet and center and maintaining a vertical posture, you're ready for the next chapter.

# Chapter Wrap-up

This chapter introduced Vertical Circles + Weight Shift, Circle #2 of our Tai Chi for Balance Exercise Set. Key takeaways include:

**The Weight Shift Powers and Controls the Vertical Circle**

- We aim for connected, whole-body movement, with the legs and hips powering and controlling the arms and hands.
- As you shift weight forward, your arms and hands extend to the Front of the Vertical Circle.
- As you shift weight back, your arms and hands bend to the Back of the Vertical Circle.
- In performing the movements, feel how your legs and hips power and control your arms and hands.

**Maintain a Vertical Posture as You Make Vertical Circles + Weight Shift**

- As you perform the movements, maintain a vertical posture, aligning the top of your head over the bottom of your pelvis.

**Honing Your Whole Body Awareness and Precise Posture Control**

- Performing Vertical Circles + Weight Shift causes constantly changing pressure in your feet. Feeling that changing pressure helps you develop increasingly consistent awareness of your feet.
- Performing Vertical Circles + Weight Shift challenges your sensitivity and skill in feeling your center and maintaining a vertical posture.
- Feeling your feet and center, and maintaining, or correcting to, a vertical posture as you move, will continue to develop your Whole Body Awareness and Precise Posture Control.

# Chapter 10

# Adding Rotation: The Hip Turn

In this chapter, we begin to explore another fundamental component of Tai Chi, **the Hip Turn**.

In Tai Chi, the Hip Turn stretches and tones the muscles and other soft tissue in and around the pelvis, upper legs, lower back, and lower abdomen. The Hip Turn also promotes circulation of blood and other fluids throughout this vital area, helping to oxygenate, nourish, and remove metabolic byproducts from the muscles, the lower digestive tract, the urinary tract, and the reproductive organs.

After getting familiar with the Hip Turn, we'll combine it with the Weight Shift, resulting in the **Weight Shift + Hip Turn**.

The Weight Shift + Hip Turn thoroughly works the muscles and connective tissues of the legs and hips, improving strength, flexibility, and circulation. When considering Tai Chi as a health practice, the Weight Shift + Hip Turn is a key component.

By strengthening the legs and hips, the Weight Shift + Hip Turn helps counteract the #1 risk factor for falling in older adults: loss of lower extremity strength. Three of the seven movements of our Tai Chi for Balance exercise set include the Weight Shift + Hip Turn.

That said, the Weight Shift + Hip Turn, requires us to pay extra attention to two sets of alignments — **our knee alignments** and what we'll call **aligning the 4 Points**. I'll cover knee alignments in this chapter and aligning the 4 Points in the next chapter.

**The importance of knee alignments**. Turning the hips can apply lateral forces and twisting forces to the knee joint. Lateral forces can collapse the knee in or out.

Twisting forces can torque the knee. These forces can aggravate existing knee conditions or cause new problems.

My experience is that most people, unless they've received knee alignment training, do **not** maintain knee alignments when turning their hips. In Tai Chi for Balance, you'll receive that training.

To that end, let's explore the Two Fundamental Knee Alignments.

## The Two Fundamental Knee Alignments

The Two Fundamental Knee Alignments are:

1. **Knee Aligned over Foot.** This means the center of the knee joint stays approximately over the center of the foot. By maintaining the knee over the foot, you'll avoid collapsing the knee in or out, and you'll avoid pushing the knee too far forward or back.

2. **Kneecap Aligned with Toes.** This means the front of the knee is facing the same direction as the foot. By keeping the kneecap aligned with the toes, you'll avoid twisting the knee.

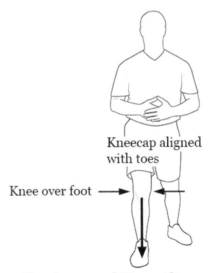

*Figure 10-1: The Two Fundamental Knee Alignments.*

**Remember our rules.** A quick review of our two rules: The 70% Rule and the Don't Cause Pain Rule. As you begin to practice the Hip Turn, move at 70% or less of your range of motion. This minimizes strain and makes it easier to maintain knee alignments. If you feel any pain in your knees while performing Hip Turns, reduce your range of motion until you can perform the Hip Turn pain-free.

With that, we proceed to another *kwa*-centered movement component that will help you maintain knee alignments while turning your hips, **the Kwa Fold**. By "Kwa Fold," I mean this: As you turn your hips into a weighted leg, by keeping the weighted leg stable, you create a diagonal crease along the front of the *kwa*. Follow my guidance, and you'll soon get a clear sense of the Kwa Fold.

## Adding Rotation: The Hip Turn + Kwa Fold

I'll start by introducing the Basic Elements of the Kwa Fold, then you'll practice it in the exercises that follow.

## Basic Elements

1. **Starting Position, Left Leg Forward Stance, weight forward**. Adjust your stance for stability and comfort. Place your hands lightly on your abdomen. Then shift weight onto your front leg. (Figure 10-2A.)

2. **Hip Turn + Kwa Fold**. Turn your hips into your weighted leg, folding into your *kwa* on that side. The Kwa Fold will help you maintain knee alignments. (Figure 10-2B.) Then turn your hips square to the front. (I call this position "hips straight ahead.") As you rotate your hips straight ahead, unfold your *kwa* and maintain your knee alignments. (Figure 10-2C.)

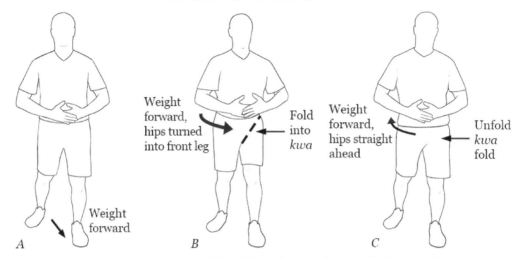

Figure 10-2: *Hip Turn + Kwa Fold, left leg forward, weight forward.*

Figure 10-3 shows two repetitions of the movement. It's not a big move. It involves a small turn of the hips into the weighted leg, then back to hips straight ahead.

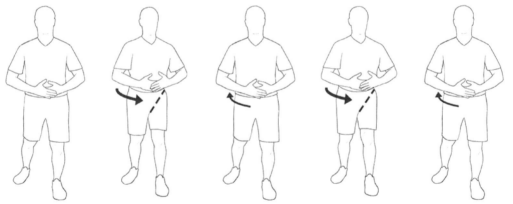

Figure 10-3: *Hip Turn + Kwa Fold, left leg forward, weight forward.*

3. **Left Leg Forward Stance, weight back.** Shift weight back, hips straight ahead. (Figure 10-4A.)

4. **Hip Turn + Kwa Fold**. Turn your hips into your weighted leg, folding into the *kwa* on that side. The Kwa Fold will help you maintain knee alignments. (Figure 10-4B.) Then turn your hips straight ahead, unfolding your *kwa*, and maintaining your knee alignments. (Figure 10-4C.)

## Adding Rotation: The Hip Turn

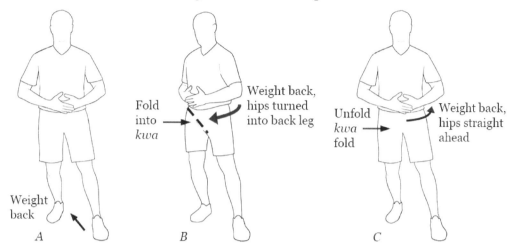

*Figure 10-4: Hip Turn + Kwa Fold, left leg forward, weight back.*

Figure 10-5 shows two repetitions of the movement.

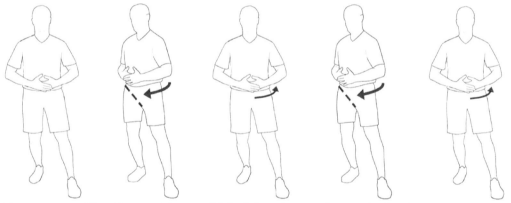

*Figure 10-5: Hip Turn + Kwa Fold, left leg forward, weight back.*

5. **Change your stance to Right Leg Forward Stance, weight forward.** Adjust your stance for stability and comfort. Then shift weight forward. (Figure 10-6A.)

6. **Hip Turn + Kwa Fold.** Turn your hips slightly into your weighted leg, folding into the *kwa* on that side. (Figure 10-6B.) Then turn your hips straight ahead, unfolding your *kwa*, and maintaining your knee alignments. (Figure 10-6C)

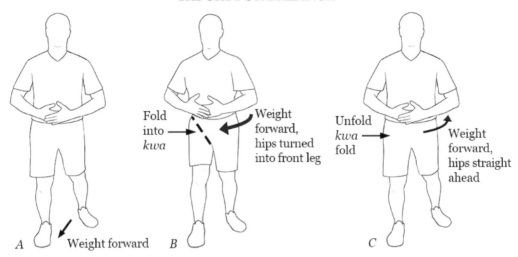

Figure 10-6: *Hip Turn + Kwa Fold, right leg forward, weight forward.*

Figure 10-7 shows two repetitions of the movement.

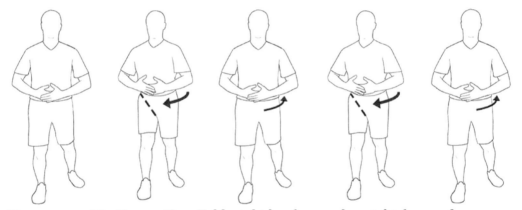

Figure 10-7: *Hip Turn + Kwa Fold, right leg forward, weight forward.*

7. **Right Leg Forward Stance, weight back.** Shift weight back, hips straight ahead. (Figure 10-8A.)

8. **Hip Turn + Kwa Fold.** Turn your hips into your weighted leg, folding into the *kwa* on that side. (Figure 10-8B.) Then turn your hips straight ahead, unfolding your *kwa*, and maintaining your knee alignments. (Figure 10-8C.)

*Adding Rotation: The Hip Turn*

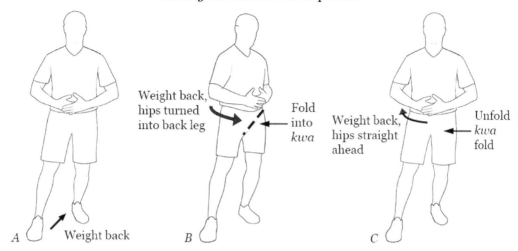

Figure 10-8: *Hip Turn + Kwa Fold, right leg forward, weight back.*

Figure 10-9 shows two repetitions of the movement.

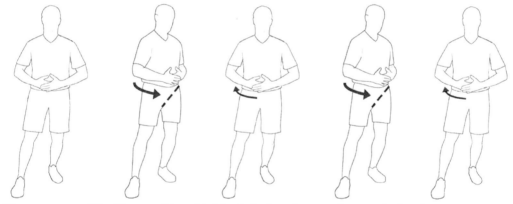

Figure 10-9: *Hip Turn + Kwa Fold, right leg forward, weight back.*

As you begin to practice the Hip Turn + Kwa Fold, I encourage you to reference the *Tips and Common Errors* in the next section. By following the tips and correcting the common errors, you will quickly discover how the Hip Turn + Kwa Fold helps you maintain your knee alignments when turning your hips.

# Tips and Common Errors

*Tips*

**Keep the Hip Turns small.** At the start, keep your Hip Turns small. Try 5 degrees past your centerline into the weighted leg. If you can maintain your knee alignments and not feel any twisting or discomfort in your knee, stick with 5 degrees for a while. On the other hand, if your knee alignments do not feel stable, or if you feel twisting or any discomfort in your knee, ***turn your hips less***. Even one degree past centerline is fine at the start.

Over time, as your knee alignments stabilize, you will find you can comfortably increase the amount of hip rotation.

**Feel your *kwa* as you fold and unfold.** In learning the Kwa Fold, it will help you to feel your *kwa*. When you do, you'll feel a gentle compression or "squish" of soft tissue as you fold into the *kwa*. As you rotate your hips away from the weighted leg and unfold your *kwa*, you will feel the gentle stretching of that soft tissue.

**Check your knee alignments frequently.** Most people, initially, do not consistently feel their knee alignments when turning their hips. I encourage you to pause frequently and check. Are your knees over your feet? Are your kneecaps aligned with your toes? Correct as needed. Practicing in front of a mirror can help.

*Common Errors*

**Not maintaining the knee over the foot.** As we turn our hips into or away from a weighted leg, correct knee alignments include aligning the knee vertically over the center of the foot—and maintaining it. A common error is allowing the knee to collapse in (Figure 10-10A) or collapse out (Figure 10-10B.)

*Adding Rotation: The Hip Turn*

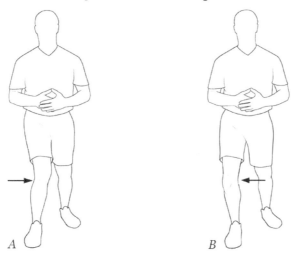

*Figure 10-10: Hip Turn + Kwa Fold, common errors, knee collapsing in or out.*

**Not maintaining the kneecap aligned with the toes.** As we turn our hips into or away from a weighted leg, correct knee alignments include aligning the kneecap with the toes—and maintaining it. That will minimize or eliminate twisting in the knee joint. A common error is allowing the kneecap to twist in (Figure 10-11A) or twist out (Figure 10-11B).

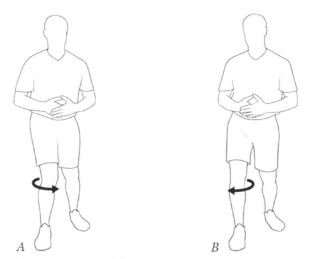

*Figure 10-11: Hip Turn + Kwa Fold, common errors, knee twisting in or out.*

With those Basic Elements, tips, and common errors in mind, let's proceed to Exercise 16 and practice the Hip Turn + Kwa Fold.

# Exercise 16: Hip Turn + Kwa Fold

1. **Getting Ready to Move.** Stand and settle into Neutral Posture. Take a minute, or more if you like, and stand quietly before moving.

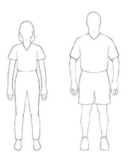

2. **Starting Position, Left Leg Forward Stance.** Adjust your stance for stability and comfort. Place your hands lightly on your abdomen. Then shift weight forward, with hips straight ahead. (Figure 10-12A)

3. **Hip Turn + Kwa Fold, weight forward, 10 repetitions.** Turn your hips into your weighted leg, fold into the *kwa* on that side. (Figure 10-12B.) Then turn your hips straight ahead, unfolding your *kwa*. (Figure 10-12C.). After each Hip Turn, check and correct your knee alignments. After 10 repetitions, turn your hips straight ahead, and shift weight back. (Figure 10-13A.)

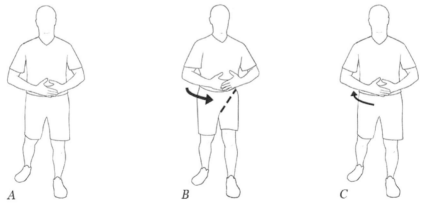

Figure 10-12: Hip Turn + Kwa Fold, left leg forward, weight forward.

4. **Hip Turn + Kwa Fold, weight back, 10 repetitions.** Turn your hips into your weighted leg, fold into the *kwa* on that side. (Figure 10-13B.) Then turn your hips

## Adding Rotation: The Hip Turn

straight ahead, unfolding your *kwa*. (Figure 10-13C.) After each Hip Turn, check and correct your knee alignments. After 10 repetitions, turn your hips straight ahead.

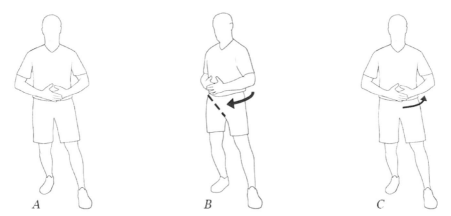

*Figure 10-13: Hip Turn + Kwa Fold, left leg forward, weight back.*

5. **Change your stance to Right Leg Forward Stance**. Shift weight forward.

6. **Hip Turn + Kwa Fold, weight forward, 10 repetitions**. (Figure 10-14A.) Turn your hips into your weighted leg, fold into the *kwa* on that side. (Figure 10-14B.). Then turn your hips straight ahead, unfolding your *kwa*. (Figure 10-14C.) After each Hip Turn, check and correct your knee alignments. After 10 repetitions, turn your hips straight ahead, and shift weight back. (Figure 10-15A.)

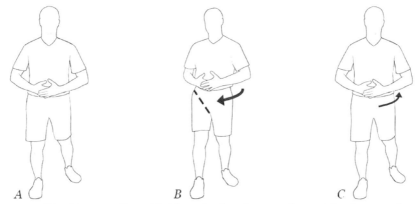

*Figure 10-14: Hip Turn + Kwa Fold, right leg forward, weight forward.*

7. **Hip Turn + Kwa Fold, weight back, 10 repetitions**. Turn your hips into your weighted leg, fold into the *kwa* on that side. (Figure 10-15B.). Then turn your hips straight ahead, unfolding your *kwa*. (Figure 10-15C.) After each Hip Turn, check and correct your knee alignments. After 10 repetitions, turn your hips straight ahead.

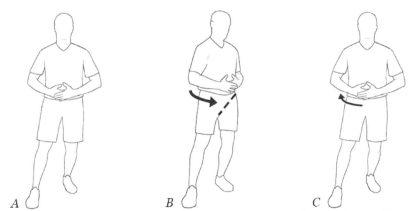

A  B  C

*Figure 10-15: Hip Turn + Kwa Fold, right leg forward, weight back.*

8. **Conclusion**. Shift your weight back. Then smoothly transition to Neutral Posture.

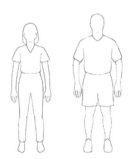

**Practice Recommendation:** Practice Exercise 16 for 1–2 days, 2–4 times each day. When you can consistently perform Hip Turns, folding into your *kwa*, and maintaining your knee alignments, you're ready for the next exercise.

It's time to add the Weight Shift. First, a short Practice Note.

*Adding Rotation: The Hip Turn*

> **Practice Note: The Weight Shift + Hip Turn and Maintaining Alignments**
>
> In the exercises that follow, you will move in increasingly dynamic ways while monitoring an increasing number of alignments. With practice, your sensitivity in feeling these alignments and your skill at maintaining or correcting them will develop. At the start, keeping it all together may seem tricky. Here are two tips that will help:
>
> **Move slowly**. For most people, moving slowly makes it easier to feel the body and monitor and correct alignments.
>
> **Pause and check.** In the beginning, I encourage you to pause frequently and check your alignments. As you develop skill in maintaining alignments while shifting your weight and turning your hips, you'll naturally begin to move more continuously and smoothly.

With that, let's proceed to the next exercise.

## Exercise 17: Weight Shift + Hip Turn

1. **Getting Ready to Move.** Stand and settle into Neutral Posture. Take a minute, or more if you like, and stand quietly before moving.

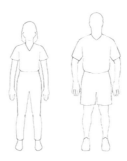

2. **Starting Position, Left Leg Forward Stance, weight back**. Adjust your stance for stability and comfort. Place your hands lightly on your abdomen. Shift weight back. Turn your hips slightly into your weighted leg. (Figure 10-16A.)

3. **Weight Shift + Hip Turn, 10 repetitions.** Smoothly shift weight forward. As you shift weight, turn your hips into the weighted leg, folding into your *kwa*.

(Figure 10-16B.) Then smoothly shift weight back, turning your hips slightly into the weighted leg, folding into your *kwa*. (Figure 10-16C.) After each weight shift + hip turn, check your knee alignments, correcting as needed. After 10 repetitions, change your stance.

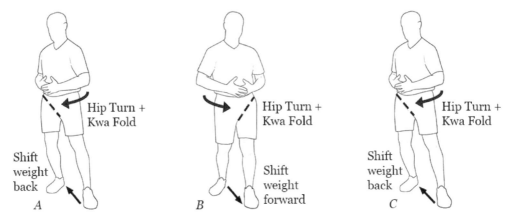

Figure 10-16: Weight Shift + Hip Turn, left leg forward.

Keeping the movements slow will help you monitor and correct your knee alignments.

4. **Right Leg Forward Stance, weight back**. Turn your hips slightly into your weighted leg, folding into your *kwa*. (Figure 10-17A.)

5. **Weight Shift + Hip Turn, 10 repetitions.** Smoothly shift weight forward. As you shift weight, turn your hips into the weighted leg, folding into your *kwa*. (Figure 10-17B.) Then smoothly shift weight back, turning your hips into the weighted leg, folding into your *kwa*. (Figure 10-17C.) After each weight shift + hip turn, check your knee alignments, correcting as needed. After 10 repetitions, shift weight back.

*Adding Rotation: The Hip Turn*

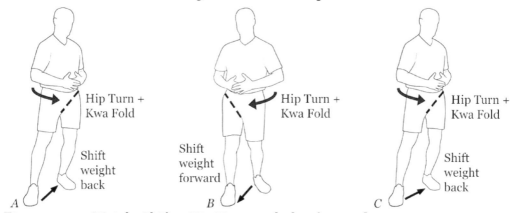

*Figure 10-17: Weight Shift + Hip Turn, right leg forward.*

6. **Conclusion**. Smoothly transition to Neutral Posture.

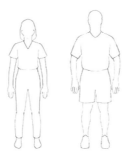

**Practice Recommendations:** Practice Exercise 17 for 1–2 days, 2–3 times each day until you can comfortably and consistently perform the Weight Shift + Hip Turn and maintain your knee alignments.

The Hip Turn raises another alignment issue: how to align the top half of the body with the bottom half of the body when turning the hips. We accomplish that by "Keeping the 4 Points Aligned." To learn how to keep your 4 Points aligned, turn to the next chapter.

# Chapter Wrap-up

This chapter introduced the Hip Turn and related movement principles and components. Key points include:

**The Two Fundamental Knee Alignments**

These are:

- Knee over foot, not collapsed in or collapsed out.
- Kneecap aligned with toes, not twisted in or twisted out.

**The Kwa Fold**

- The Kwa Fold helps us maintain our knee alignments as we turn our hips into a weighted leg.
- When we turn our hips into a weight leg, we fold into the kwa on the weighted side.
- As we turn our hips back to straight ahead, we unfold the kwa.

**The Weight Shift + Hip Turn**

- The Weight Shift + Hip Turn combines the forward and back movement of the Weight Shift with the rotational movement of the Hip Turn.
- The following techniques will help you develop skill in maintaining the Two Fundamental Knee Alignments while shifting weight and turning your hips:
    - Feeling your knees
    - Moving slowly and smoothly
    - Incorporating the Kwa Fold
    - Pausing frequently to check knee alignments, correcting as needed

# Chapter 11

## Adding Rotation: Keeping the 4 Points Aligned

The previous chapter focused on knee alignments, a key to stabilizing the lower body and protecting your knees when turning the hips. This chapter covers how we connect the upper half of the body to the lower half of the body when turning the hips. For that, we incorporate a principle called **Keeping the 4 Points Aligned**.

## Your 4 Points and How to Keep Them Aligned

First, we need to find our 4 Points. We already found the lower 2 Points back in Chapter 5. The lower 2 Points are the front of the *kwa* on our left and right sides (Figure 11-1.)

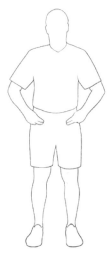

*Figure 11-1: Finding your 4 Points, the lower 2 Points.*

The upper 2 points are located on each side of the torso, approximately in front of the shoulder joint. We'll call these points the **Shoulder's Nests**.

**Finding your Shoulder's Nests.** I encourage you to find your Shoulder's Nests and feel them with your fingers. You want to develop a clear awareness of these areas of your body. Try the following procedure in front of a mirror.

To find your right Shoulder's Nest, take the index and middle fingers of your left hand and find your sternum—the flat bone in the center of your chest. At the top of your sternum, you will feel a U-shaped notch (the *suprasternal notch*). Then find your right clavicle—the long, thin bone extending horizontally from the top of your sternum to your right shoulder. Then walk your fingers out toward your shoulder to the end of your clavicle.

At the end of your clavicle, you'll feel a joint (the *acromioclavicular joint*, or "AC joint"). From the AC joint, walk your fingers back along the clavicle about an inch. Then drop your fingers down just below the clavicle. There you will find an indentation, a "nest" below the bone and between the muscles of the chest and shoulder. When you press it, it will feel soft, even squishy. That's your right Shoulder's Nest. (Figure 11-2A.)

To find your left Shoulder's Nest, repeat the procedure on your left side. (Figure 11-2B.)

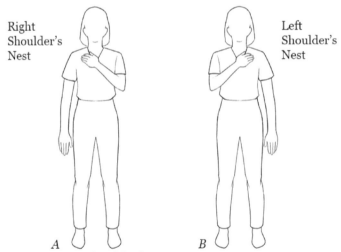

*Figure 11-2: Finding your Shoulder's Nests.*

Now you have the upper 2 Points. Add those to your lower 2 Points, and you've found your 4 Points. (Figure 11-3.)

## Adding Rotation: Keeping the 4 Points Aligned

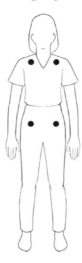

*Figure 11-3: The 4 Points.*

**Aligning the 4 Points.** After finding the 4 Points, we are now ready to align them. In front of the mirror, find your right Shoulder's Nest with your left hand. With your right hand, find the center of your *kwa* on your right side. (Figure 11-4A.) Note the vertical orientation of these two parts of your body. The right Shoulder's Nest is located along a vertical line, directly above the center of your kwa on the right side. Next, find your left Shoulder's Nest and the center of your kwa on the left side. (Figure 11-4B.) Again, note the vertical orientation of these two parts of your body.

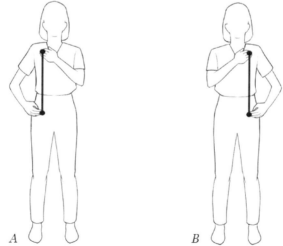

*Figure 11-4: Vertical alignment of Shoulder's Nests and kwa.*

Next, settle into Neutral Posture. When each Shoulder's Nest is directly above the corresponding point on the front of the *kwa*, the 4 Points form a rectangle. As we move in Tai Chi, including when we turn our hips, we aim to maintain this rectangle. We call this **Keeping the 4 Points Aligned**. (Figure 11-5.)

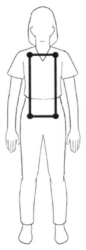

*Figure 11-5: Keeping the 4 Points Aligned.*

**Feel when your 4 Points are aligned.** I encourage you to stand for a minute or two, feeling how it feels to align your 4 Points. Your shoulders are directly over your hips. Your spine is not twisted.

**Feel when the 4 Points are *not* aligned.** Next, keeping your hips straight ahead, move one shoulder forward and the other shoulder back. Note how your Shoulder's Nests are no longer directly above the corresponding point on the front of the *kwa*. Your 4 Points are *not* aligned. Note the sensation of twisting in your spine.

**Keeping the 4 Points Aligned.** We want to keep the rectangle made by our 4 Points intact. Put another way, all the rotation comes from the legs and hips. The upper half of the body rides along above the pelvis, turning as the hips turn.

A new concept for you? That's normal. Most people new to Tai Chi have no experience in Keeping the 4 Points Aligned. People are not used to rotating the upper body solely from the hips and legs. It's common to rotate the body by leading with the arms, shoulders, or head. When leading rotation with the arms, shoulders, or head, the spine twists. When the spine twists, the 4 Points are *not* aligned.

*Adding Rotation: Keeping the 4 Points Aligned*

Within limits, most bodies twist without a problem. But it is not the connected, whole-body movement of Tai Chi. When we rotate in Tai Chi, we connect the bottom and top halves of the body by Keeping the 4 Points Aligned.

Exercise 18 will help you develop the sensitivity and skill to keep your 4 Points Aligned.

## Exercise 18: Weight Shift + Hip Turn + Keeping the 4 Points Aligned

1. **Getting Ready to Move.** Stand and settle into Neutral Posture. Take a minute, or more if you like, and stand quietly before moving.

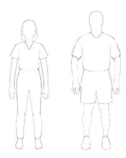

2. **Starting Position, Left Leg Forward Stance.** Adjust your stance for stability and comfort. Place your hands lightly on your abdomen. Shift weight back. Turn your hips into your weighted leg, folding into the *kwa*. (Figure 11-6A.)

3. **Check your alignments**. Align your Shoulder's Nests vertically over the corresponding points on the front of your *kwa*. Check your knee alignments too. Knee over foot, kneecap aligned with toes.

4. **Weight Shift + Hip Turn, 10 repetitions.** Smoothly shift weight forward, turning your hips into the weighted leg, folding into the *kwa*. (Figure 11-6B.) Then smoothly shift weight back, turning your hips into the weighted leg, folding into the *kwa*. (Figure 11-6C.) Check your 4 Points and knee alignments, correcting as needed. After 10 repetitions, shift weight back. (Figure 11-7A.)

5. **Change your stance to Right Leg Forward Stance**. Shift weight back. Turn your hips into your weighted leg, folding into the *kwa*.

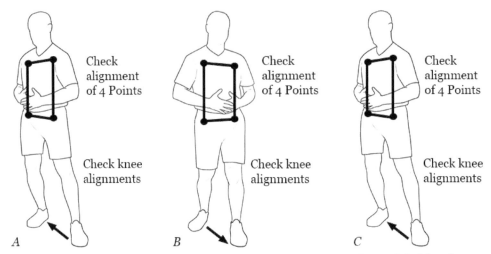

Figure 11-6: Weight Shift + Hip Turn + Keeping the 4 Points Aligned, left leg forward.

6. **Weight Shift + Hip Turn, 10 repetitions.** Shift weight back. Turn your hips into the weighted leg. Smoothly shift weight forward, turning your hips into the weighted leg, folding into the *kwa*. (Figure 11-7B.) Then smoothly shift weight back, turning your hips into the weighted leg, folding into the *kwa*. (Figure 11-7C.) Check your 4 Points and knee alignments, correcting as needed. After 10 repetitions, shift weight back.

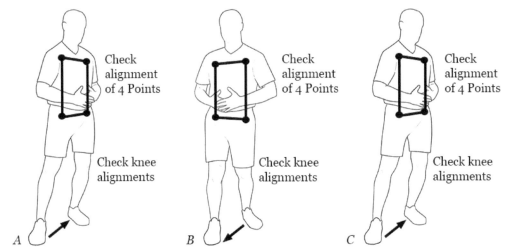

Figure 11-7: Weight Shift + Hip Turn + Keeping the 4 Points Aligned, right leg forward.

7. **Conclusion.** Smoothly transition to Neutral Posture.

*Adding Rotation: Keeping the 4 Points Aligned*

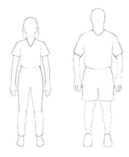

**Practice Recommendations:** Exercise 18 builds upon the alignment skills from Chapter 10, extending your awareness from your knees through your *kwa* to your shoulders. In doing so, you'll move your body in an increasingly connected manner. You're also keeping track of more "moving parts," continuing to develop your Whole Body Awareness.

I recommend practicing Exercise 18 for 1–2 days, 2–4 times each day. When you can perform the Weight Shift + Hip Turn while consistently Keeping the 4 Points Aligned and maintaining knee alignments, you're ready for the next exercise.

In Exercise 19, you'll refine your Whole Body Awareness, developing skill at maintaining multiple alignments and feeling your feet and center, all while performing dynamic, multiplane motion.

For most of us, this can seem tricky at first. There's a lot to keep track of. With the skills you've developed so far, plus a little practice, you'll soon get the hang of it.

# Exercise 19: Weight Shift + Hip Turn + Feeling Your Feet and Center

For the movements of Exercise 19, you can reference the instructions and figures for Exercise 18.

**Practice Video.** You can also follow me in the guided practice video covering this exercise. To access the video, go to https://www.chicagotaichi.org/tai-chi-for-balance-guided-practice-videos/

1. **Getting Ready to Move.** Take a minute, or more if you like, and stand quietly before moving. First, settle into Neutral Posture. Then feel your feet, balancing the pressure in your feet. Then feel your center, aligning your center vertically.

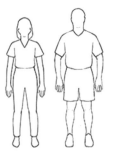 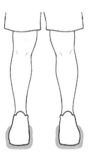 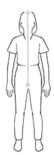

2. **Starting Position, Left Leg Forward Stance**. Shift weight back. Place your hands lightly on your abdomen. Turn your hips into your weighted leg, folding into the *kwa*.

3. **Weight Shift + Hip Turn, 10 repetitions**. Smoothly shift weight forward, turning your hips into the weighted leg, folding into the *kwa*. Then smoothly shift weight back, turning your hips into the weighted leg, folding into your *kwa*. With each Weight Shift + Hip Turn, feel your feet, maintain a vertical center, and check your alignments, correcting as needed. After 10 repetitions, shift weight back.

4. **Change your stance to Right Leg Forward Stance**. Shift weight back. Turn your hips into your weighted leg, folding into the *kwa*.

5. **Weight Shift + Hip Turn, 10 repetitions**. Smoothly shift weight forward, turning your hips into the weighted leg, folding into the *kwa*. Then smoothly shift

*Adding Rotation: Keeping the 4 Points Aligned*

weight back, turning your hips into the weighted leg, folding into your *kwa*. Feel your feet, center, and alignments as described above, correcting as needed. After 10 repetitions, shift weight back.

6. **Conclusion**. Smoothly transition to Neutral Posture.

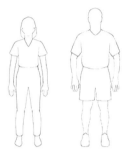

**Practice Recommendation:** Exercise 19 may feel like a step up. Lots to feel, monitor, and adjust. With practice, your sensitivity and skill will increase, and it will take less conscious effort to keep all the alignments in place. Practice Exercise 19 for 1–3 days, 2–4 times each day. When you can perform the Weight Shift + Hip Turn while:

- Keeping the 4 Points Aligned
- Maintaining the Two Fundamental Knee Alignments
- Feeling the constantly changing pressures in your feet, and
- Maintaining a vertical posture

you're ready for the next chapter.

Now, it's time to add more moving parts—the arms!

# Chapter Wrap-up

This chapter introduced Keeping the 4 Points Aligned, a core alignment principle when we add rotation. Key points include:

**Keeping the 4 Points Aligned**

- The 4 Points consist of the center of the front of the *kwa* on the right and left side (the lower 2 Points) and the Shoulder's Nests on the front of each shoulder (the upper 2 Points).
- The 4 Points form a rectangle. Keeping the 4 Points Aligned means maintaining that rectangle as we move.
- With the 4 Points aligned, the shoulders are aligned above the pelvis and the spine is not twisted.
- With the 4 Points aligned, we move the pelvis, torso, neck, and head as a connected unit.
- It is common to lead rotational movement with the arms and shoulders. This twists the spine and misaligns the 4 points. In Tai Chi, the rotation comes from the legs and the hips.

**Continuing to develop Whole Body Awareness and Precise Posture Control**

- In performing the Weight Shift + Hip Turn while feeling your feet and center, you monitor an increasing number of body parts, alignments, and sensations.
- Moving slowly and smoothly and, initially, pausing after each Weight Shift + Hip Turn to check and correct your alignments, will help you develop the necessary sensitivity and skill. Soon your movements will become smooth and continuous.
- Developing the Whole Body Awareness and Precise Posture control necessary to perform the movements, maintain your alignments, feel your feet, and feel your center is a key objective in the Tai Chi for Balance System. In doing so, you'll maintain a more stable, fall-resistant structure.

# Chapter 12

## Circle #3: Vertical Circles + Weight Shift + Hip Turn

We now have the movement components and alignments we need to introduce Circle #3: Vertical Circles + Weight Shift + Hip Turn.

For starters, Circle #3 is low-impact, yet powerful exercise. Regular practice of Circle #3:

- ➢ Strengthens, stretches, and improves circulation in the entire lower half of the body.
- ➢ Stretches, releases tension, and improves circulation in the entire upper half of the body.
- ➢ Trains the nervous system to coordinate smooth, connected, whole-body movement, powering and controlling the top half of the body from the bottom half of the body.

As part of the Tai Chi for Balance System, practicing Vertical Circles + Weight Shift + Hip Turn sharpens your sensitivity and skills in maintaining Whole Body Awareness and developing increasingly Precise Posture Control—all while performing dynamic, multiplane movements.

At the start, most people find Circle #3 challenging to coordinate. Not to worry. I'll guide you through a process that's helped thousands of students and clients become proficient in Circle #3. Just follow my instructions in this chapter. Soon, you'll perform Circle #3 as smooth, connected, whole-body movement.

We'll begin with the Basic Elements.

## Basic Elements

1. **Starting Position, Left Leg Forward Stance.** Shift weight back. Turn your hips into the weighted leg. Place your hands at the Back of your Vertical Circle. (Figure 12-1.) We'll start with Top to Bottom Vertical Circles.

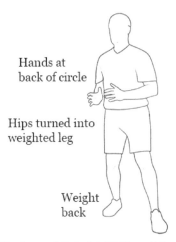

*Figure 12-1: Vertical Circles + Weight Shift + Hip Turn, left leg forward, Starting Position.*

2. **Top of Vertical Circle.** Shift half your weight forward, turning your hips straight ahead, as you extend your arms and your hands to the Top of your Vertical Circle. (Figure 12-2A.)

3. **Front of Vertical Circle.** Shift weight fully forward, turning your hips into the front leg as you extend your arms and hands to the Front of your Vertical Circle. (Figure 12-2B.)

*Circle #3: Vertical Circles + Weight Shift + Hip Turn*

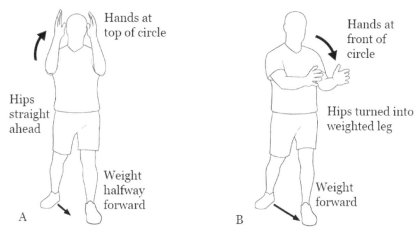

*Figure 12-2: Vertical Circles + Weight Shift + Hip Turn, left leg forward, Top and Front of Vertical Circle.*

4. **Bottom of Vertical Circle.** Shift half your weight back, turning your hips straight ahead as you bend your arms and circle your hands to the Bottom of your Vertical Circle. (Figure 12-3A.)

5. **Back of Vertical Circle.** Shift weight fully back, turning your hips into your back leg, as you bend your arms and circle your hands to the Back of your Vertical Circle. (Figure 12-3B.)

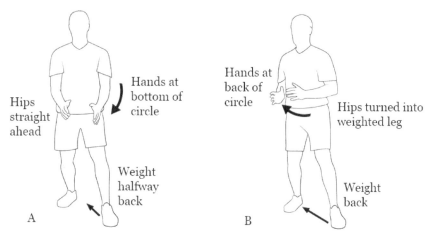

*Figure 12-3: Vertical Circles + Weight Shift + Hip Turn, left leg forward, Bottom and Back of Vertical Circle.*

Figure 12-4 shows those movements in sequence.

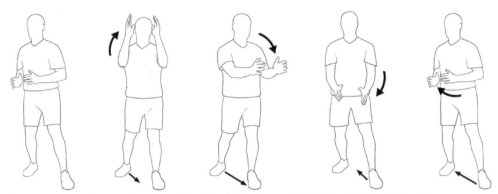

*Figure 12-4: Top to Bottom Vertical Circles + Weight Shift + Hip Turn, left leg forward.*

6. **Change directions**. Make Bottom to Top Vertical Circles.

7. **Bottom of Vertical Circle**. From the Back of your Vertical Circle, shift half your weight forward, turning your hips straight ahead as you extend your arms and hands to the Bottom of your Vertical Circle. (Figure 12-5A.)

8. **Front of Vertical Circle.** Shift weight fully forward, turning your hips into your front leg as you extend your arms and hands to the Front of your Vertical Circle. (Figure 12-5B.)

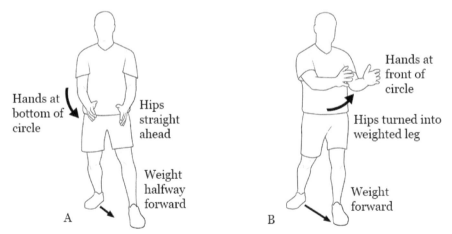

*Figure 12-5: Vertical Circles + Weight Shift + Hip Turn, left leg forward, Bottom and Front of Vertical Circle.*

*Circle #3: Vertical Circles + Weight Shift + Hip Turn*

9. **Top of Vertical Circle.** Shift half your weight back, turning your hips straight ahead as you bend your arms and circle your hands to the Top of your Vertical Circle. (Figure 12-6A.)

10. **Back of Vertical Circle.** Shift weight fully back, turning your hips into your back leg as you bend your arms and circle your hands to the Back of your Vertical Circle. (Figure 12-6B.)

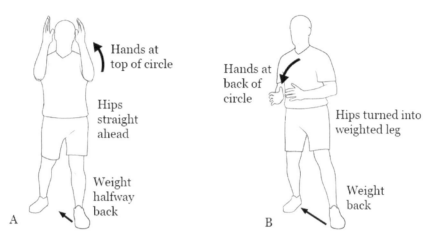

Figure 12-6: Vertical Circles + Weight Shift + Hip Turn, left leg forward, Top and Back of Vertical Circle.

Figure 12-7 shows those movements in sequence.

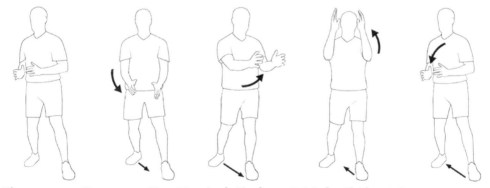

Figure 12-7: Bottom to Top Vertical Circles + Weight Shift + Hip Turn, left leg forward.

11. **Change your stance to Right Leg Forward Stance.** Shift weight back, turning your hips into the weighted leg. Position your hands at the Back of your Vertical Circle. (Figure 12-8.) After changing stances, we'll begin with Top to Bottom Vertical Circles.

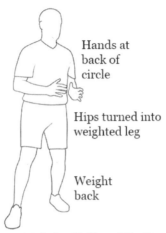

Figure 12-8: *Vertical Circles + Weight Shift + Hip Turn, right leg forward, Starting Position.*

12. **Top of Vertical Circle.** Shift half your weight forward, turning your hips straight ahead as you extend your arms and hands to the Top of your Vertical Circle. (Figure 12-9A.)

13. **Front of Vertical Circle.** Shift weight fully forward, turning your hips into your front leg as you extend your arms and hands to the Front of your Vertical Circle. (Figure 12-9B.)

## Circle #3: Vertical Circles + Weight Shift + Hip Turn

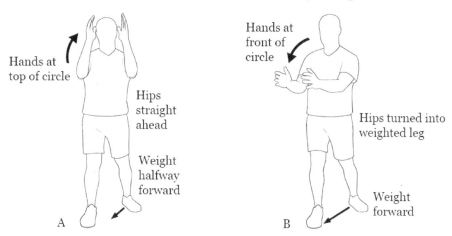

Figure 12-9: *Vertical Circles + Weight Shift + Hip Turn, right leg forward, Top and Front of Vertical Circle.*

14. **Bottom of Vertical Circle.** Shift half your weight back, turning your hips straight ahead as you bend your arms and circle your hands to the Bottom of your Vertical Circle. (Figure 12-10A.)

15. **Back of Vertical Circle.** Shift weight fully back, turning your hips into your back leg as you bend your arms and circle your hands to the Back of your Vertical Circle. (Figure 12-10B.)

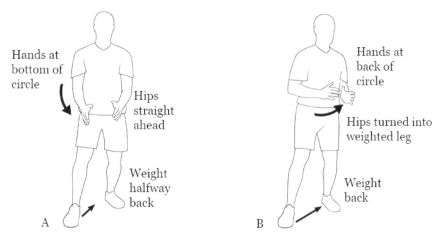

Figure 12-10: *Vertical Circles + Weight Shift + Hip Turn, right leg forward, Bottom and Back of Vertical Circle.*

Figure 12-11 shows those movements in sequence.

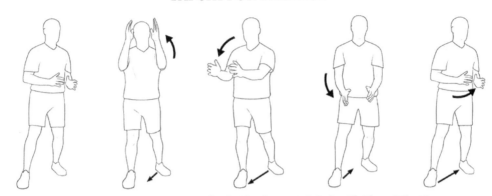

*Figure 12-11: Top to Bottom Vertical Circles + Weight Shift + Hip Turn, right leg forward.*

16. **Change directions.** Make Bottom to Top Vertical Circles.

17. **Bottom of Vertical Circle.** From the Back of your Vertical Circle, shift half your weight forward, turning your hips straight ahead as you extend your arms and hands to the Bottom of your Vertical Circle. (Figure 12-12A.)

18. **Front of Vertical Circle.** Shift weight fully forward, turning your hips into your front leg as you extend your arms and hands to the Front of your Vertical Circle. (Figure 12-12B.)

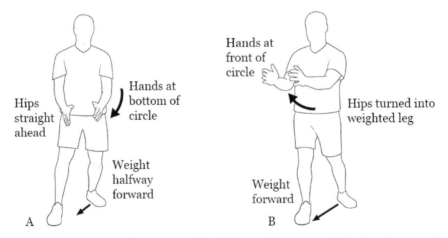

*Figure 12-12: Vertical Circles + Weight Shift + Hip Turn, right leg forward, Bottom and Front of Vertical Circle.*

## Circle #3: Vertical Circles + Weight Shift + Hip Turn

19. **Top of Vertical Circle.** Shift half your weight back, turning your hips straight ahead, as you bend your arms and circle your hands to the Top of your Vertical Circle. (Figure 12-13A.)

20. **Back of Vertical Circle.** Shift weight fully back, turning your hips into your back leg as you bend your arms and circle your hands to the Back of your Vertical Circle. (Figure 12-13B.)

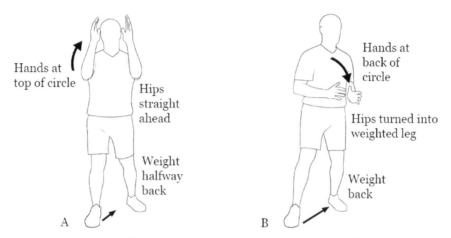

Figure 12-13: Vertical Circles + Weight Shift + Hip Turn, right leg forward, Top and Back of Vertical Circle.

Figure 12-14 shows those movements in sequence.

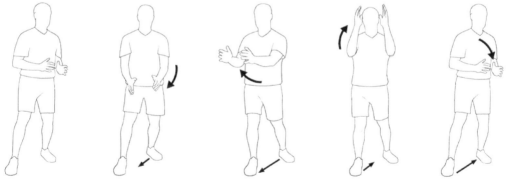

Figure 12-14: Bottom to Top Vertical Circles + Weight Shift + Hip Turn, right leg forward.

If that seems like a lot to absorb, I empathize. Initially, most people find Vertical Circles + Weight Shift + Hip Turn challenging to put together.

In teaching sophisticated movement for years to a wide range of learners, I've developed a go-to learning strategy for moves like Circle #3. It goes like this:

- **Break the move into parts**
- **Pause at each part**
- **Check**
- **Correct**

For most people, following this approach results in rapidly developing the necessary coordination to perform Circle #3 smoothly and accurately.

Let's turn to that now.

## Learning Circle #3: The Four Checkpoints

To follow this learning strategy, we break each Vertical Circle into four parts or "checkpoints"—the Back, the Bottom, the Front, and the Top. I recommend you pause briefly at each checkpoint, check several elements, correcting as necessary. Here's how you do it, starting with Top to Bottom Vertical Circles + Weight Shift + Hip Turn.

**Part 1 –Back of Vertical Circle.** This is the starting point and the point you return to for transitioning, either when changing directions or changing stances.

What to check (Figure 12-15):

- ✓ Weight on back leg
- ✓ Hips rotated into back leg, folding into the kwa
- ✓ Hands approximately a fist's distance away from torso, positioned at Back of Vertical Circle
- ✓ Basic alignments set: Tailbone relaxed down, midriff open, occiput lifted, head over pelvis, and torso vertical (not leaning)
- ✓ 4 Points Aligned: Shoulders aligned over pelvis, spine not twisted
- ✓ Knees aligned: Knee over respective foot, not collapsed in or out; kneecap aligned with respective toes, not twisted in or out

*Circle #3: Vertical Circles + Weight Shift + Hip Turn*

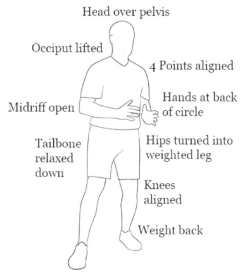

*Figure 12-15: Vertical Circle + Weight Shift + Hip Turn, checking the Back of your Vertical Circle.*

Now let's move to the Top of your Vertical Circle.

**Part 2 –Top of Vertical Circle**

What to check (Figure 12-16):

- ✓ Weight even between back and front legs
- ✓ Hips straight ahead
- ✓ Hands at Top of Vertical Circle
- ✓ Basic alignments set
- ✓ 4 Points aligned
- ✓ Knees aligned

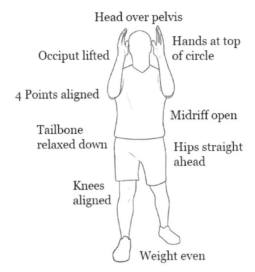

*Figure 12-16: Vertical Circle + Weight Shift + Hip Turn, checking the Top of your Vertical Circle.*

Now let's move to the Front of your Vertical Circle.

## Part 3 – Front of Vertical Circle

What to check (Figure 12-17):

- ✓ Weight on front leg
- ✓ Hips turned into front leg, folding into the *kwa*
- ✓ Hands at Front of Vertical Circle
- ✓ Elbows slightly bent, not locked
- ✓ Basic alignments set
- ✓ 4 Points aligned
- ✓ Knees aligned

### Circle #3: Vertical Circles + Weight Shift + Hip Turn

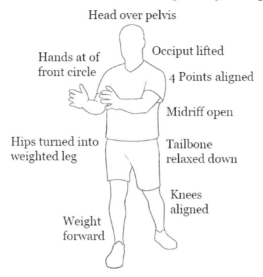

Figure 12-17: Vertical Circle + Weight Shift + Hip Turn, checking the Front of your Vertical Circle.

Now let's move to the Bottom of your Vertical Circle.

## Part 4 –Bottom of Vertical Circle

What to check (Figure 12-18):

- ✓ Weight even between the back and front legs
- ✓ Hips straight ahead
- ✓ Hands at Bottom of Vertical Circle
- ✓ Basic alignments set
- ✓ 4 Points are aligned
- ✓ Knees aligned

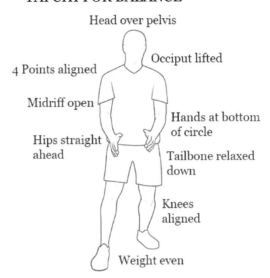

*Figure 12-18: Vertical Circle + Weight Shift + Hip Turn, checking the Bottom of your Vertical Circle.*

When you've completed all four movements, return to the Back of your Vertical Circle.

**Changing directions.** When you perform Bottom to Top Vertical Circles + Weight Shift + Hip Turn, the four parts go like this:

Part 1 – Back of Vertical Circle
Part 2 – Bottom of Vertical Circle
Part 3 – Front of Vertical Circle
Part 4 – Top of Vertical Circle

At each checkpoint, use the applicable checklist. Follow the same procedure after changing stances.

After practicing Circle #3 slowly, pausing at each checkpoint, and correcting as necessary, your movements will soon become increasingly smooth, connected, and accurate.

With that, let's proceed to Exercise 20.

*Circle #3: Vertical Circles + Weight Shift + Hip Turn*

# Exercise 20: Vertical Circles + Weight Shift + Hip Turn

1. **Getting Ready to Move.** Stand and settle into Neutral Posture. Take a minute, or more if you like, and stand quietly before moving.

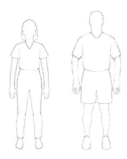

2. **Starting Position, Left Leg Forward.** Shift weight back. Turn your hips into your weighted leg. Place your hands at the Back of your Vertical Circle. (Figure 12-19A.)

3. **Make Top to Bottom Vertical Circles, 5 repetitions.** Smoothly shift weight forward, turning your hips into your front leg as you extend your arms and hands through the Top and Front of your Vertical Circle. (Figure 12-19B-C.) Then smoothly shift weight back, turning your hips into your back leg as you bend your arms and circle your hands through the Bottom and Back of your Vertical Circle. (Figure 12-19D-E.) After 5 repetitions, return to the Back of your Vertical Circle.

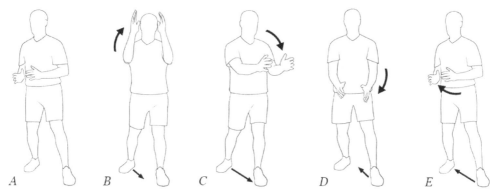

*Figure 12-19: Top to Bottom Vertical Circles + Weight Shift + Hip Turn, left leg forward.*

4. **Change directions; make Bottom to Top Vertical Circles.** Smoothly shift weight forward, turning your hips into your front leg as you extend your arms and hands through the Bottom and Front of your Vertical Circle. (Figure 12-20B-C.) Then smoothly shift weight back, turning your hips into your back leg as you bend your arms and circle your hands through the Top and Back of your Vertical Circle. (Figure 12-20D-E.) After 5 repetitions, return to the Back of your Vertical Circle.

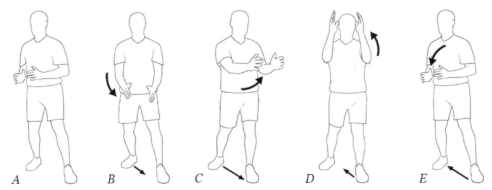

*Figure 12-20: Bottom to Top Vertical Circles + Weight Shift + Hip Turn, left leg forward.*

5. **Change your stance to Right Leg Forward Stance.** Shift weight back. Position your hands at the Back of your Vertical Circle. (Figure 12-21A.)

6. **Make Top to Bottom Vertical Circles, 5 repetitions.** Smoothly shift weight forward, turning your hips into your front leg as you extend your arms your hands through the Top and Front of your Vertical Circle. (Figure 12-21B-C.) Then smoothly shift weight back, turning your hips into your back leg as you bend your arms and circle your hands through the Bottom and Back of your Vertical Circle. (Figure 12-21D-E.) After 5 repetitions, return to the Back of your Vertical Circle.

*Circle #3: Vertical Circles + Weight Shift + Hip Turn*

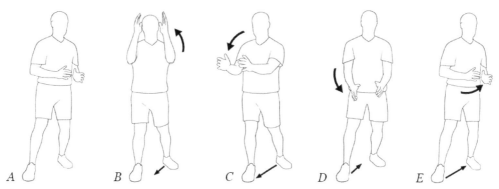

Figure 12-21: *Top to Bottom Vertical Circles + Weight Shift + Hip Turn, right leg forward.*

7. **Change directions; make Bottom to Top Vertical Circles, 5 repetitions**. Smoothly shift weight forward, turning your hips into your front leg as you extend your arms and hands through the Bottom and Front of your Vertical Circle. (Figure 12-22B-C.) Then smoothly shift weight back, turning your hips into your back leg as you bend your arms and circle your hands through the Top and Back of your Vertical Circle. (Figure 12-22D-E.) After 5 repetitions, return to the Back of your Vertical Circle.

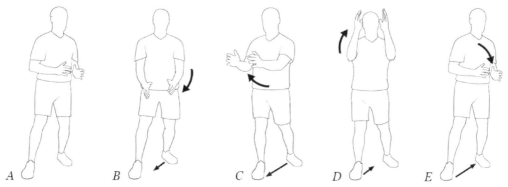

Figure 12-22: *Bottom to Top Vertical Circles + Weight Shift + Hip Turn, right leg forward.*

8. **Conclusion**. Smoothly transition to Neutral Posture.

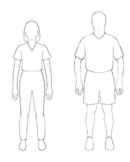

**Practice Recommendation:** Practice Exercise 20 for 2–4 days, 2–3 times each day. When you can comfortably perform a set of 20 Vertical Circles + Weight Shifts + Hip Turns, you're ready for the next exercise. It's time to add feeling your feet and center.

## Exercise 21: Vertical Circles + Weight Shift + Hip Turn + Feeling Your Feet and Center

For the movements of Exercise 21, you can reference the instructions and figures accompanying Exercise 20.

**Practice Video.** You can also follow me in the guided practice video covering this exercise. To access the video, go to https://www.chicagotaichi.org/tai-chi-for-balance-guided-practice-videos/

1. **Getting Ready to Move.** Take a minute, or more if you like, and stand quietly before moving. First, settle into Neutral Posture. Then feel your feet, balancing the pressure in your feet. Then feel your center, aligning your center vertically.

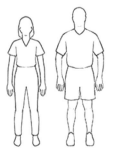 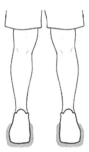 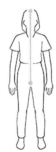

*Circle #3: Vertical Circles + Weight Shift + Hip Turn*

2. **Starting Position, Left Leg Forward Stance**. Shift weight back. Turn your hips slightly into your weighted leg. Place your hands at the Back of your Vertical Circle.

3. **Make Top to Bottom Vertical Circles, 5 repetitions**. As you move, feel your feet. Feel the constantly changing pressure in each foot. Feel your center. Maintain, or correct to, a vertical posture. After 5 repetitions, return to the Back of your Vertical Circle.

4. **Change directions, make Bottom to Top Vertical Circles**. As you move, feel your feet and center as described above. After 5 repetitions, return to the Back of your Vertical Circle.

5. **Change your stance to Right Leg Forward Stance**. Shift weight back. Position your hands at the Back of your Vertical Circle.

6. **Make Top to Bottom Vertical Circles, 5 repetitions.** As you move, feel your feet and center as described above. After 5 repetitions, return to the Back of your Vertical Circle.

7. **Change directions, make Bottom to Top Vertical Circles, 5 repetitions.** As you move, feel your feet and center as described above. After 5 repetitions, return to the Back of your Vertical Circle.

8. **Conclusion**. Smoothly transition to Neutral Posture.

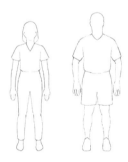

**Practice Recommendation:** Practice Exercise 21 for 2–4 days, 2–3 times each day. When you can comfortably make a set of 20 Vertical Circles + Weight Shifts + Hip Turns, while feeling your feet and maintaining, or correcting to, a vertical posture, you're ready for the next chapter. It's time for a set of Circles #1–#3.

# Chapter Wrap-up

This chapter introduced Circle #3: Vertical Circles + Weight Shift + Hip Turn. Initially, most people find Circle #3 challenging to coordinate. With a little practice, you'll get it just fine.

Key points include:

**Learning Circle #3, the 4 Checkpoints**

- I recommend breaking down Circle #3 into 4 Checkpoints: the Back, Top, Front, and Bottom of the Vertical Circle.
- At each checkpoint, pause and check the following, correcting as needed:
    - Where your weight is
    - Your hip position
    - Your hand position
    - Your postural alignments
    - Your knee alignments
    - Your 4 Points
- For most of us, that's a lot to keep track of. Pausing at each checkpoint, and checking and correcting your "moving parts" will help you coordinate the movement.

**Honing Your Whole Body Awareness and Precise Posture Control**

- Performing Vertical Circles + Weight Shift + Hip Turn causes constantly changing pressure in each foot. Feeling that changing pressure will help you develop increasingly consistent awareness of your feet.
- Maintaining, or correcting to, a vertical posture during the movement will increase your sensitivity to feeling your center and will refine your skill at Precise Posture Control.
- All of this contributes to developing a more stable, fall-resistant structure while performing increasingly dynamic movement.

# Chapter 13

## Building Our Tai Chi for Balance Exercise Set: Circles #1 through #3

At this point, you've practiced much of the core material in the Tai Chi for Balance System. This includes:

- The 70% Rule
- The Don't Cause Pain Rule
- Neutral Posture
- Feeling Your Feet
- Feeling Your Center
- The Kwa Squat
- Vertical Circles
- Circle #1: Vertical Circles + Kwa Squat
- The Weight Shift
- Circle #2: Vertical Circles + Weight Shift
- The Hip Turn
- The Kwa Fold
- The Two Fundamental Knee Alignments
- Keeping the 4 Points Aligned
- The Weight Shift + Hip Turn
- Circle #3: Vertical Circles + Weight Shift + Hip Turn
- Feeling your feet and center while performing increasingly dynamic movement
- Maintaining a vertical posture, except when intentionally inclining the torso

That's a lot! Plus, much of the material is new. Feel good about your progress!

By now, you're on the path to achieving the three main Tai Chi for Balance objectives:

- ➢ Developing Whole Body Awareness
- ➢ Developing Precise Posture Control
- ➢ Developing strong legs and hips

With practice, the strength, skill, and sensitivity you're developing will **keep you on your feet and out of the emergency room**.

Now, it's time to begin to build our movement set, Tai Chi Circling Hands. We'll start by performing Circles #1 through #3 in sequence. A full set includes 20 repetitions of each movement, including direction changes and stance changes.

With that, let's go to Exercise 22.

# Exercise 22: Circles #1 through #3

The following instructions guide you step-by-step through a full set of Circles #1 through #3.

**Practice Video.** You can also follow me in the guided practice video covering this exercise. To access the video, go to https://www.chicagotaichi.org/tai-chi-for-balance-guided-practice-videos/

**Getting Ready to Move**

Take a minute, or more if you like, and stand quietly before moving.

- ➤ Settle into Neutral Posture.
- ➤ Feel your feet, balancing the pressure in your feet.
- ➤ Feel your center, aligning your center vertically.

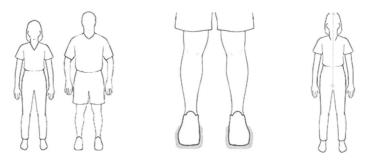

**Circle #1: Vertical Circles + Kwa Squat**

1. **Circle #1 Starting Position**. Sink into a Kwa Squat. Place your hands at the Back of your Vertical Circle. (Figure 13-1A.) Feel for any pressure changes in your feet. Feel your center inclined slightly forward.

2. **Make Top to Bottom Vertical Circles, 10 repetitions**. (Figure 13-1A-E). As you move, feel your feet and center. Before and after each Kwa Squat, balance the pressures in your feet and return your center to the vertical. After 10 repetitions, return to the Back of your Vertical Circle.

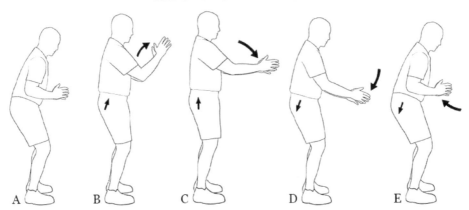

*Figure 13-1: Circle #1, Top to Bottom Vertical Circles + Kwa Squat.*

3. **Change directions; make Bottom to Top Vertical Circles, 10 repetitions.** (Figure 13-2A-E). As you move, feel your feet and center as described above. After 10 repetitions, return to the Back of your Vertical Circle. Proceed to Circle #2 Starting Position.

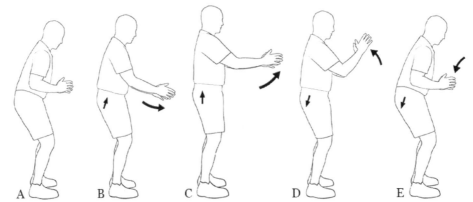

*Figure 13-2: Circle #1, Top to Bottom Vertical Circles + Kwa Squat.*

## Circle #2: Vertical Circles + Weight Shift

1. **Starting Position, Left Leg Forward Stance**. Shift weight back. Place your hands at the Back of your Vertical Circle. (Figure 13-3A.) Feel your feet; one loaded, one unloaded. Feel your center. Establish a vertical posture.

2. **Make Top to Bottom Vertical Circles, 5 repetitions.** (Figure 13-3A-E.) As you move, feel your feet. Feel the constantly changing pressure in each foot. Feel

your center. Maintain, or correct to, a vertical posture. After 5 repetitions, return to the Back of your Vertical Circle.

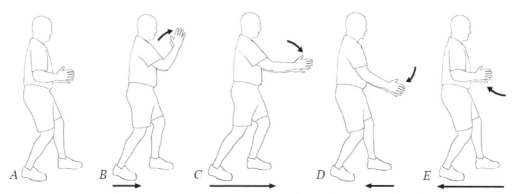

Figure 13-3: Circle #2, Top to Bottom Vertical Circles + Weight Shift, left leg forward.

3. **Change directions, make Bottom to Top Vertical Circles, 5 repetitions**. (Figure 13-4A-E.) As you move, feel your feet and center as described above. After 5 repetitions, return to the Back of your Vertical Circle.

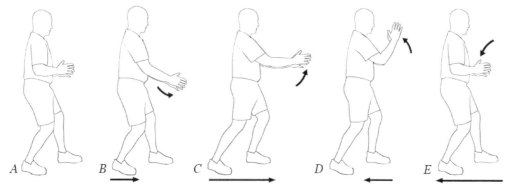

Figure 13-4: Circle #2, Bottom to Top Vertical Circles + Weight Shift, left leg forward.

4. **Change your stance to Right Leg Forward Stance**. Shift weight back. Place your hands at the Back of your Vertical Circle. (Figure 13-5A.)

5. **Make Top to Bottom Vertical Circles, 5 repetitions**. (Figure 13-5A-E.) As you move, feel your feet and center as described above. After 5 repetitions, return to the Back of your Vertical Circle.

TAI CHI FOR BALANCE

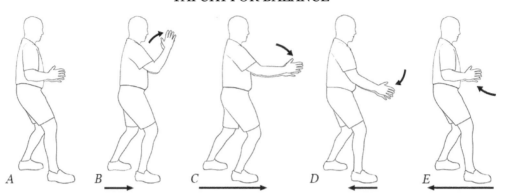

*Figure 13-5: Circle #2, Top to Bottom Vertical Circles + Weight Shift, right leg forward.*

6. **Change directions; make Bottom to Top Vertical Circles, 5 repetitions**. (Figure 13-6A-E.) As you move, feel your feet and center as described above. After 5 repetitions, return to the Back of your Vertical Circle. Then go to Circle #3 Starting Position.

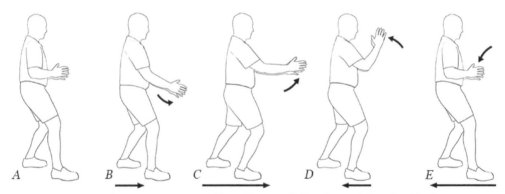

*Figure 13-6: Circle #2, Bottom to Top Vertical Circles + Weight Shift, right leg forward.*

### Circle #3: Vertical Circles + Weight Shift + Hip Turn

1. **Starting Position, Left Leg Forward Stance**. Shift weight back. Turn your hips into your weighted leg. Place your hands at the Back of your Vertical Circle. (Figure 13-7A.) Feel your feet; one loaded, one unloaded. Feel your center. Establish a vertical posture.

*Building Our Tai Chi for Balance Exercise Set: Circles #1 through #3*

2. **Make Top to Bottom Vertical Circles, 5 repetitions.** (Figure 13-7A-E.) As you move, feel your feet. Feel the constantly changing pressure in each foot. Feel your center. Maintain, or correct to, a vertical posture. After 5 repetitions, return to the Back of your Vertical Circle.

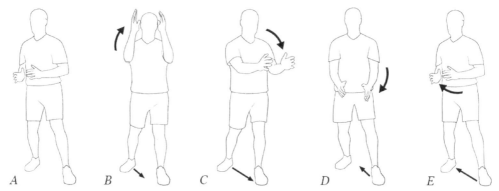

*Figure 13-7: Circle #3, Top to Bottom Vertical Circles + Weight Shift + Hip Turn, left leg forward.*

3. **Change directions; make Bottom to Top Vertical Circles, 5 repetitions**. (Figure 13-8A-E.) As you move, feel your feet and center as described above. After 5 repetitions, return to the Back of your Vertical Circle.

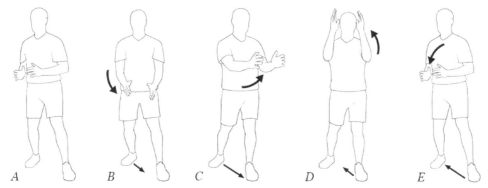

*Figure 13-8: Circle #3, Bottom to Top Vertical Circles + Weight Shift + Hip Turn, left leg forward.*

4. **Change your stance to Right Leg Forward Stance**. Shift weight back. Turn your hips into your weighted leg. Position your hands at the Back of your Vertical Circle. (Figure 13-9A.)

5. **Make Top to Bottom Vertical Circles, 5 repetitions**. (Figure 13-9A-E.) As you move, feel your feet and center as described above. After 5 repetitions, return to the Back of your Vertical Circle.

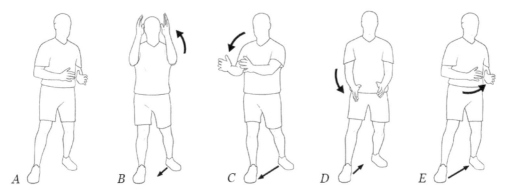

Figure 13-9: Circle #3, Top to Bottom Vertical Circles + Weight Shift + Hip Turn, right leg forward.

6. **Change directions; make Bottom to Top Vertical Circles, 5 repetitions**. (Figure 13-10A-E.) As you move, feel your feet as described above. After 5 repetitions, return to the Back of your Vertical Circle.

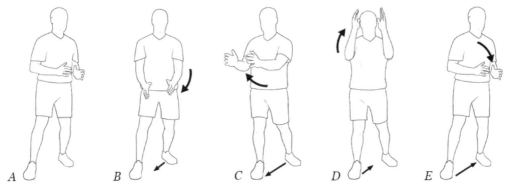

Figure 13-10: Circle #3, Bottom to Top Vertical Circles + Weight Shift + Hip Turn, right leg forward.

## Conclusion

> **Smoothly return to Neutral Posture**.

*Building Our Tai Chi for Balance Exercise Set: Circles #1 through #3*

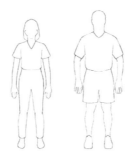

> **Stand in Neutral Posture for 1–2 minutes**. Notice how you feel after 60 circles, 20 Kwa Squats, 80 Weight Shifts, and 40 Hip Turns. That's a growing volume of low-impact exercise, all while practicing Whole Body Awareness and Precise Posture Control with increasing sensitivity and skill.

**Practice Recommendation:** Practice Exercise 22 for 2–3 days, 1–2 times each day. When you can comfortably perform a full set of Circles #1 through #3, proceed to Part 3. It's time to change the plane of our circles.

# Part 3

# Continuing to Move:

# Horizontal Circles

In Part 3, we build upon all the previous material, adding Circle #4: Horizontal Circles + Kwa Squat and Circle #5: Horizontal Circles + Weight Shift + Hip Turn. Besides changing the plane of the circles, nearly all other movement components are familiar—the Kwa Squat, the Weight Shift + Hip Turn, maintaining alignments, feeling your feet, and feeling your center. For Horizontal Circles, we add another component to the Kwa Squat—small hip turns. By now, you've built a solid foundation for incorporating that.

Separated into three short chapters, Part 3 moves quickly. By the end, you'll progress to 20 repetitions each of Circles #1 through #5, increasing the volume of your Tai Chi for Balance workout.

Let's turn to the next chapter and begin exploring Horizontal Circles.

# Chapter 14

## Circle #4: Horizontal Circles + Kwa Squat

In Part 2, we used Vertical Circles to explore a fundamental characteristic of Tai Chi movements—circularity. For Circles #4 and #5, we continue exploring circular movement, changing the plane of our circles from vertical to horizontal (also called the "transverse plane").

Circular movement is a key to many of Tai Chi's proven health benefits. For example, the circular movements of the arms in Tai Chi gently stretch and relax your shoulders, upper back, and neck. Similarly, the hip rotation added to the Kwa Squat and in the Weight Shift + Hip Turn helps these movements work into tight spots in the hips, legs, lower back, and abdomen. As chronic tension eases, the muscles and associated soft tissue become more relaxed and mobile. Circulation of blood and other fluid improves. Tightness, aches, and pains subside.

By changing our arm and hand movements to Horizontal Circles, we change the direction of the stretch and release in and around the shoulders and upper back. This works the joints, muscles, and other soft tissues from different angles, helping to relax and release more tight areas.

As part of the Tai Chi for Balance System, Horizontal Circles change the patterns of pressure in the feet and the forces affecting our posture. By adding Horizontal Circles to our movements, we further develop our Whole Body Awareness and Precise Posture Control.

**Practice Note: Clockwise and Counterclockwise Circles**

As an exercise physiologist and Tai Chi instructor, I am trained to analyze, describe, and teach human movement. That includes linear movement (in a straight line) and rotational or angular movement (circling around a point). In describing the *direction* of rotational movement, I follow the convention of using "counterclockwise" and "clockwise." These terms are based on how the hands move around the face of an *analog* clock. In a world dominated by *digital* clocks, a quick Practice Note might help.

**Counterclockwise** means rotating in the *opposite* direction of the hands of a clock, like this:

**Clockwise** means rotating in the *same* direction as the hands of a clock, like this:

When I use these terms, I am referring to the direction of the circle from the perspective of the *person performing the movement.*

For the direction of Horizontal Circles, assume the clock is lying flat in front of you.

If "counterclockwise" and "clockwise" ever leaves you unsure about the direction to make circles, don't worry. Just pick a direction and make circles in that direction. When my instructions say, "change directions," circle the other way.

*Circle #4: Horizontal Circles + Kwa Squat*

Let's turn now to the Basic Elements of Horizontal Circles + Kwa Squat.

# Basic Elements

1. **Starting Position**. Sink into a Kwa Squat, with your hips straight ahead. Bend your arms and place your hands in front of your torso, palms facing down, approximately a fist's distance away from your body. Pick a comfortable height for your hands. For example, the level of your diaphragm. This is the Back of your Horizontal Circle. (Figure 14-1.) We'll begin by making counterclockwise Horizontal Circles.

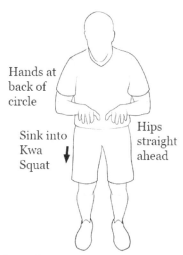

*Figure 14-1: Horizontal Circles + Kwa Squat, Starting Position.*

2. **Right Side of Horizontal Circle**. From the Starting Position, begin rising out of your Kwa Squat and turning your hips to your right as you extend your arms slightly, beginning to move your hands away from the body. Turning the hips combined with extending the arms moves the hands to the Right Side of your Horizontal Circle. (Figure 14-2A.)

3. **Front of Horizontal Circle**. From the Right Side of your Horizontal Circle, rise fully out of your Kwa Squat, turning your hips from your right to straight ahead as you stretch your arms, moving your hands further away from the body. Continue until your hips are straight ahead and your arms and hands are in front of you. This is the Front of your Horizontal Circle. (Figure 14-2B.)

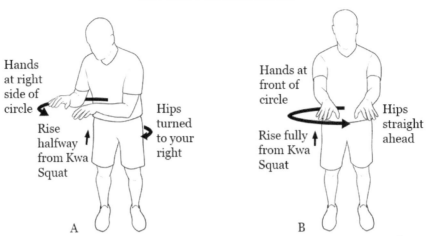

Figure 14-2: *Counterclockwise Horizontal Circles + Kwa Squat, Right Side and Front of Horizontal Circle.*

4. **Left Side of the Horizontal Circle.** From the Front of your Horizontal Circle, begin to sink into a Kwa Squat, turning your hips to your left as you bend your arms slightly, beginning to move the hands toward the body. Turning the hips to the left combined with bending the arms moves your hands to the Left Side of your Horizontal Circle. (Figure 14-3A.)

5. **Back of Horizontal Circle.** From the Left Side of your Horizontal Circle, sink fully into a Kwa Squat, turning your hips from your left to straight ahead as you bend your arms, moving your hands back toward the body. Continue until you are at the bottom of your Kwa Squat, with your hips, arms, and hands straight ahead. You have returned to the Back of your Horizontal Circle. (Figure 14-3B.)

*Circle #4: Horizontal Circles + Kwa Squat*

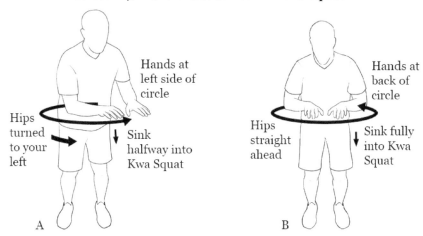

Figure 14-3: *Counterclockwise Horizontal Circles + Kwa Squat, Left Side and Back of Horizontal Circle.*

Figure 14-4 shows the movements in sequence.

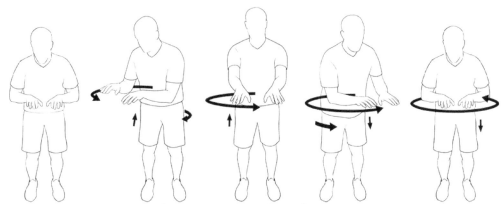

Figure 14-4: *Counterclockwise Horizontal Circles + Kwa Squat.*

6. **Change directions.** We now change the direction of hip rotation, making clockwise Horizontal Circles.

7. **Left Side of Horizontal Circle.** From the Back of your Horizontal Circle, begin rising out of your Kwa squat, turning your hips to your left as you extend your arms, beginning to move your hands away from the body. Turning the hips combined with extending the arms moves the hands to the Left Side of your Horizontal Circle. (Figure 14-5A.)

8. **Front of Horizontal Circle.** From the Left Side of your Horizontal Circle, rise fully out of your Kwa Squat, turning your hips from to your left to straight ahead as you stretch your arms, moving your hands further away from the body. Continue until your hips are straight ahead and your arms and hands are extended in front of you. This is the Front of your Horizontal Circle. (Figure 14-5B.)

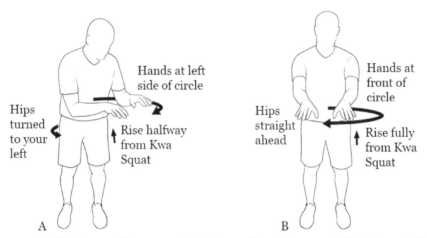

*Figure 14-5: Clockwise Horizontal Circles + Kwa Squat, Left Side and Front of Horizontal Circle.*

9. **Right Side of Horizontal Circle.** From the Front of your Horizontal Circle, begin to sink into a Kwa Squat, turning your hips to your right as you bend your arms slightly, beginning to move the hands toward the body. Turning the hips to the right combined with bending the arms moves your hands to the Right Side of your Horizontal Circle. (Figure 14-6A.)

10. **Back of Horizontal Circle.** From the Right Side of your Horizontal Circle, continue to sink into a Kwa Squat, turning your hips from your right to straight ahead as you bend your arms, moving your hands back toward the body. Continue until you are at the bottom of your Kwa Squat, with your hips, arms, and hands straight ahead. You have returned to the Back of your Horizontal Circle. (Figure 14-6B.)

### Circle #4: Horizontal Circles + Kwa Squat

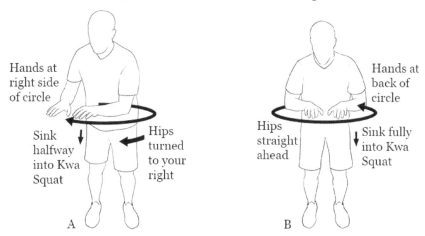

Figure 14-6: *Clockwise Horizontal Circles + Kwa Squat, Right Side and Back of Horizontal Circle.*

Figure 14-7 shows the movements in sequence.

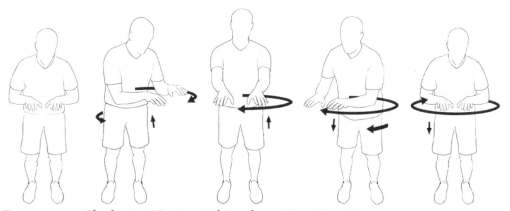

Figure 14-7: *Clockwise Horizontal Circles + Kwa Squat.*

As you begin to practice Horizontal Circles + Kwa Squat, I recommend you reference the *Tips and Common Errors* next section. Following the tips and correcting the common errors helps most people perform smooth, accurate Horizontal Circles in short order.

# Tips and Common Errors

*Tips*

**Make Horizontal Circles by turning the hips as you perform Kwa Squats, plus bending and stretching the arms.** To move the arms and hands toward the body, sink into a Kwa Squat as you bend your arms. To move the arms and hands away from the body, rise out of a Kwa Squat and stretch your arms. To make the arms and hands circle to the right or left, rotate the hips in the desired direction. Combining these movement components results in the hands tracing Horizontal Circles. The arms and hands generally stay oriented in front of the torso, extending to the Front of the Horizontal Circle and bending to the Back of the Horizontal Circle.

**Pick a height for your hands, keeping them at that height.** Choose a comfortable height for your hands and aim to keep them at that height as you circle. In the beginning, the specific height you choose is not important. Later, you can experiment with different heights for your hands. Changing the height of the hands changes the areas in your back that are stretched by the movements, helping you to target different tight spots.

**Keep the movements relaxed.** The Horizontal Circle + Kwa Squat does *not* involve tensing the shoulders, arms, hands, or any other body part. By releasing tension and relaxing, you will find it easier to perform smooth, continuous, circular movements.

**Feel your back, shoulders, and neck.** As you perform the movements, feel your back, shoulders, and neck. As the arms extend, feel for a light stretch in those areas. As the arms bend, feel for a gentle release. With practice, the sensations of stretching and releasing become smooth and continuous as you circle.

*Common Errors*

**Making circles by twisting the spine.** It is common for people initially to make Horizontal Circles by twisting their spine rather than turning their hips. This breaks the alignment of the 4 Points. You want to keep your spine neutral, your 4 Points aligned, moving your hands around the circle mainly by turning your hips. (Figure 14-8A.)

*Circle #4: Horizontal Circles + Kwa Squat*

**Locking the elbows at the front of the circle.** The 70% Rule applies. A common error when extending the arms is extending too much, locking the elbows. This induces tension. (Figure 14-8B.)

**Tensing the hands and fingers.** Through all our movements, we want to keep our hands relaxed. A common error is tensing the hands and fingers. (Figure 14-8B.)

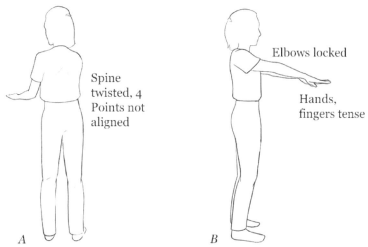

Figure 14-8: Horizontal Circles + Kwa Squat, common errors.

With those Basic Elements, tips, and commons errors as guidance, let's proceed to Exercise 23.

# Exercise 23: Horizontal Circles + Kwa Squat

1. **Getting Ready to Move.** Stand and settle into Neutral Posture. Take a minute, or more if you like, and stand quietly before moving.

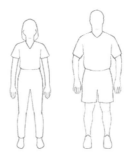

2. **Starting Position.** Sink into a Kwa Squat, hips straight ahead. Place your hands at the Back of your Horizontal Circle. (Figure 14-9A.)

3. **Make counterclockwise Horizontal Circles, 10 repetitions.** From the Starting Position, rise out of your Kwa Squat, turning your hips as you extend your arms and circle your hands through the Right Side and Front of your Horizontal Circle. (Figure 14-9B-C.) Then sink into a Kwa Squat, turning your hips as you bend your arms and circle your hands through the Left Side and Back of your Horizontal Circle. (Figure 14-9D-E.) After 10 repetitions, return to the Back of your Horizontal Circle.

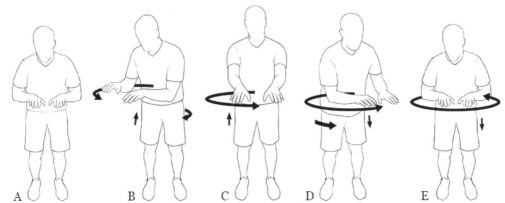

*Figure 14-9: Counterclockwise Horizontal Circles + Kwa Squat.*

*Circle #4: Horizontal Circles + Kwa Squat*

4. **Change directions; make clockwise Horizontal Circles, 10 repetitions.** From the Back of your Horizontal Circle (Figure 14-10A), rise out of a Kwa Squat, turning your hips as you extend your arms and circle your hands through the Left Side and Front of your Horizontal Circle. (Figure 14-10B-C.) Then sink into your Kwa Squat, turning your hips, as you bend your arms and circle your hands through the Right Side and Back of your Horizontal Circle. (Figure 14-10D-E.) After 10 repetitions, return to the Back of your Horizontal Circle.

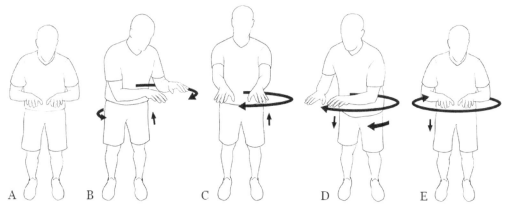

Figure 14-10: *Clockwise Horizontal Circles + Kwa Squat.*

5. **Conclusion.** Smoothly transition to Neutral Posture.

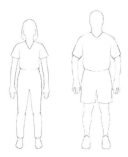

**Practice Recommendation:** Practice Exercise 23 for 1–2 days, 2–4 times each day. When you can comfortably make a set of 20 Horizontal Circles + Kwa Squats, you're ready for the next exercise. It's time to add feeling your feet and center.

TAI CHI FOR BALANCE

# Exercise 24: Horizontal Circles + Kwa Squat + Feeling Your Feet and Center

For the movements of Exercise 24, you can reference the instructions and figures accompanying Exercise 23.

**Practice Video.** You can also follow me in the guided practice video covering this exercise. To access the video, go to https://www.chicagotaichi.org/tai-chi-for-balance-guided-practice-videos/

1. **Getting Ready to Move.** Take a minute, or more if you like, and stand quietly before moving. First, settle into Neutral Posture. Then feel your feet, balancing the pressure in your feet. Then feel your center, aligning your center vertically.

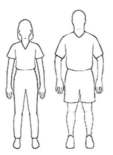 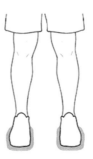 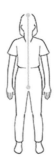

2. **Starting Position.** Sink into a Kwa Squat, hips straight ahead. Place your hands at the Back of your Horizontal Circle.

3. **Make counterclockwise Horizontal Circles, 10 repetitions.** As you move, feel your feet and center. Before and after each Kwa Squat, balance the pressures in your feet and return your center to the vertical. After 10 repetitions, return to the Back of your Horizontal Circle.

4. **Change directions; make clockwise Horizontal Circles, 10 repetitions.** As you move, feel your feet and center as described above. After 10 repetitions, return to the Back of your Horizontal Circle.

5. **Conclusion.** Smoothly transition to Neutral Posture.

*Circle #4: Horizontal Circles + Kwa Squat*

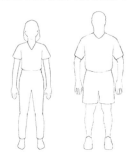

**Practice Recommendation:** Practice Exercise 23 for 1–2 days, 2–4 times each day. When you can comfortably make a set of 20 Horizontal Circles + Kwa Squats, while feeling your feet and center, you're ready for the next chapter.

## Chapter Wrap-up

This chapter introduced Circle #4, Horizontal Circles + Kwa Squat. Here's a summary of key points.

### Make Horizontal Circles by Coordinating the Kwa Squat, Hip Turns, and Bending and Stretching the Arms

- We make Horizontal Circles mainly with the action of the legs and hips, plus the bending and stretching of the arms.
- Sinking into the Kwa Squat and bending the arms brings the hands to Back of the Horizontal Circle.
- Rising from Kwa Squat and stretching the arms sends the hands to the Front of the Horizontal Circle.
- The hip turns move the hands around the Horizontal Circle.

### Continuing to Develop Whole Body Awareness and Precise Posture Control

- Performing Horizontal Circles + Kwa Squats results in different patterns of pressure in your feet and different forces affecting your posture.
- Balancing the pressures in your feet and feeling your center as you move will help you continue to develop Whole Body Awareness and Precise Posture Control.

# Chapter 15

## Circle #5: Horizontal Circles + Weight Shift + Hip Turn

For our next movement, Circle #5, we add the Weight Shift + Hip Turn, putting more leg and hip action into our Horizontal Circles. Practicing Circle #5 will continue to:

- Strengthen, stretch, and improve circulation in the entire lower half of the body.
- Stretch, release tension, and improve circulation in the entire upper half of the body.
- Train the nervous system to coordinate smooth, connected, whole-body movement, with the body half of the body powering and controlling the top half of the body.

Compared to Circles #1–#4, Circle #5 generates different forces going through your feet and affecting your posture. As part of the Tai Chi for Balance System, Circle #5 helps you hone your Whole Body Awareness and Precise Posture Control—all while performing dynamic, multiplane movement.

With that, let's proceed to the Basic Elements of Circle #5.

## Basic Elements

1. **Starting Position, Left Leg Forward Stance**. Adjust your stance for stability and comfort. Shift weight back. Turn your hips into your weighted leg. Place your hands at the Back of your Horizontal Circle. (Figure 15-1.) We'll begin by making counterclockwise Horizontal Circles.

# TAI CHI FOR BALANCE

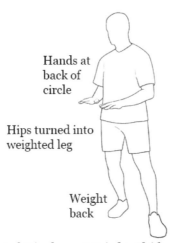

Figure 15-1: Horizontal Circles + Weight Shift + Hip Turn, left leg forward, Starting Position.

2. **Front of Horizontal Circle**. From the Starting Position, shift weight forward, as you turn your counterclockwise hips toward your front leg. At the same time, extend your arms as you circle your hands counterclockwise to the Front of your Horizontal Circle. (Figure 15-2A.) Coordinate your movements so you complete the Weight Shift + Hip Turn as your hands reach the Front of the Horizontal Circle.

3. **Back of Horizontal Circle.** Then shift weight back, as you turn your hips counterclockwise toward your back leg. At the same time, bend your arms as you circle your hands counterclockwise to the Back of your Horizontal Circle. (Figure 15-2B.) Coordinate your movements so you complete the Weight Shift + Hip Turn as your hands reach the Back of the Horizontal Circle.

*Circle #5: Horizontal Circles + Weight Shift + Hip Turn*

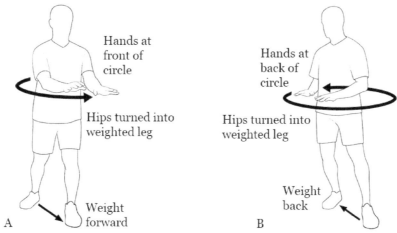

Figure 15-2: Counterclockwise Horizontal Circles + Weight Shift + Hip Turn, left leg forward, Front and Back of Horizontal Circle.

Figure 15-3 shows two repetitions of this movement.

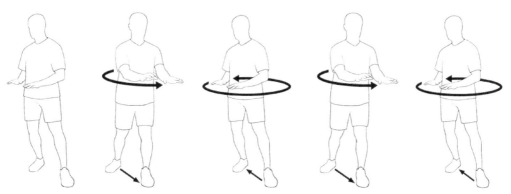

Figure 15-3: Counterclockwise Horizontal Circles + Weight Shift + Hip Turn, left leg forward.

4. **Change directions.** Starting from the Back of your Horizontal Circle (Figure 15-4), change the direction of your Horizontal Circles to clockwise.

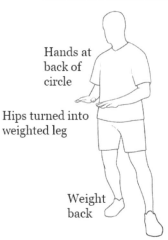

*Figure 15-4: Clockwise Horizontal Circles + Weight Shift + Hip Turn, left leg forward, Back of Horizontal Circle.*

5. **Front of the Horizontal Circle.** Shift weight forward, as you turn your hips clockwise toward your front leg. At the same time, extend your arms as you circle your hands clockwise to the Front of your Horizontal Circle. (Figure 15-5A.) Coordinate your movements so you complete the Weight Shift + Hip Turn as your hands reach the Front of the Horizontal Circle.

6. **Back of Horizontal Circle.** Then shift weight back, as you turn your hips clockwise toward your back leg. At the same time, bend your arms as you circle your hands clockwise to the Back of your Horizontal Circle. (Figure 15-5B.) Coordinate your movements so you complete the Weight Shift + Hip Turn as your hands reach the Back of the Horizontal Circle.

## Circle #5: Horizontal Circles + Weight Shift + Hip Turn

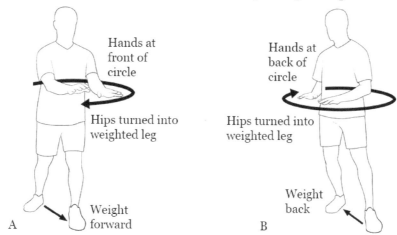

Figure 15-5: Clockwise Horizontal Circles + Weight Shift + Hip Turn, left leg forward, Front and Back of Horizontal Circle.

Figure 15-6 shows two repetitions of this movement.

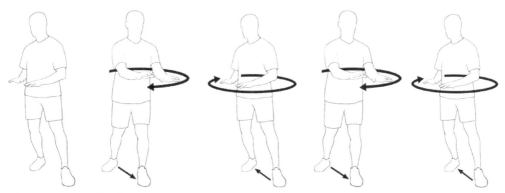

Figure 15-6: Clockwise Horizontal Circles + Weight Shift + Hip Turn, left leg forward.

7. **Change your stance to Right Leg Forward Stance**. Shift weight back, turning your hips into the weighted leg. Place your hands at the Back of your Horizontal Circle. (Figure 15-7.) With the right leg forward, we begin with clockwise Horizontal Circles.

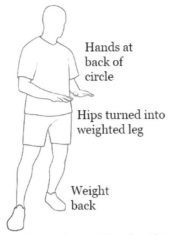

*Figure 15-7: Clockwise Horizontal Circles + Weight Shift + Hip Turn, right leg forward, Back of Horizontal Circle.*

8. **Front of Horizontal Circle**. Shift weight forward, as you turn your hips clockwise toward your front leg. At the same time, extend your arms as you circle your hands clockwise to the Front of your Horizontal Circle. (Figure 15-8A.) Coordinate your movements so you complete the Weight Shift + Hip Turn as your hands reach the Front of the Horizontal Circle.

9. **Back of Horizontal Circle.** Then shift weight back, as you turn your hips clockwise toward your back leg. At the same time, bend your arms as you circle your hands toward your torso, returning to the Back of your Horizontal Circle. (Figure 15-8B.) Coordinate your movements so you complete the Weight Shift + Hip Turn as your hands reach the Back of the Horizontal Circle.

*Circle #5: Horizontal Circles + Weight Shift + Hip Turn*

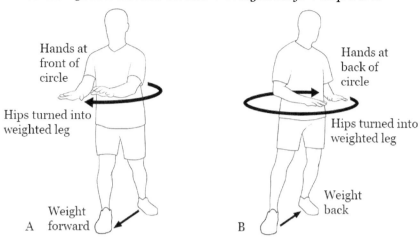

Figure 15-8: Clockwise Horizontal Circles + Weight Shift + Hip Turn, right leg forward, Front and Back of Horizontal Circle.

Figure 15-9 shows two repetitions of this movement.

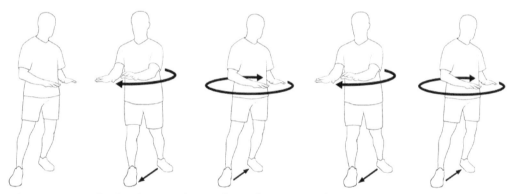

Figure 15-9: Clockwise Horizontal Circles + Weight Shift + Hip Turn, right leg forward.

10. **Change directions.** From the Back of your Horizontal Circle, change the direction of your Horizontal Circles to counterclockwise.

11. **Front of Horizontal Circle.** Shift weight forward, as you rotate your hips counterclockwise toward your front leg. At the same time, stretch your arms as you circle your hands counterclockwise to the Front of your Horizontal Circle. (Figure 15-10A.) Coordinate your movements so you complete the Weight Shift + Hip Turn as your hands reach the Front of the Horizontal Circle.

12. **Back of Horizontal Circle.** Shift weight back, as you turn your hips clockwise toward your back leg. At the same time, bend your arms as you circle your hands toward your torso, returning to the Back of your Horizontal Circle. (Figure 15-10B.) Coordinate your movements so you complete the Weight Shift + Hip Turn as the hands reach the Back of the Horizontal Circle.

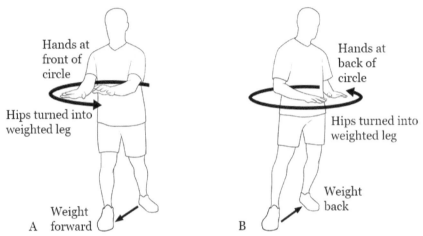

*Figure 15-10: Counterclockwise Horizontal Circles + Weight Shift + Hip Turn, right leg forward, Front and Back of Horizontal Circle.*

Figure 15-11 shows two repetitions of this movement.

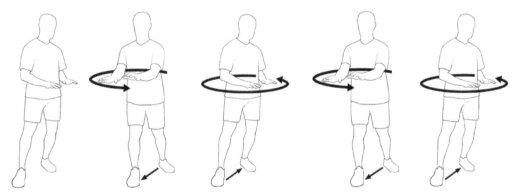

*Figure 15-11: Counterclockwise Horizontal Circles + Weight Shift + Hip Turn, right leg forward.*

## Circle #5: Horizontal Circles + Weight Shift + Hip Turn

As you begin to practice Circle #5, I encourage you to review the *Tips and Common Errors* in the next section. By following the tips and correcting common errors, you'll soon perform the movements in an increasingly smooth and connected manner.

## Tips and Common Errors

*Tips*

**Make Horizontal Circles by turning the hips and shifting weight, plus bending and stretching the arms.** To make the arms and hands circle counterclockwise or clockwise, turn the hips in the desired direction. To move the arms and hands away from the body, shift the weight forward while extending the arms. To bring the arms and hands back toward the body, shift the weight back while bending the arms. The arms and hands generally stay oriented in front of the torso, extending to reach the Front of the Horizontal Circle and bending to return to the Back of the Horizontal Circle.

**Balance the size of your Horizontal Circle with the size of your Weight Shift + Hip Turn.** If your Weight Shifts + Hip Turns are small, make small Horizontal Circles. You are aiming for connected, balanced, whole-body movement.

*Common Errors*

**Leading with the arms and hands.** A common error is to lead the turning with the hands, arms, and shoulders. This twists the spine, breaking the alignment of the 4 Points. (Figure 15-12A.)

**Arms pulling the torso forward.** When shifting weight forward and extending the arms, a common error is to lean forward. (Figure 15-12B.)

# TAI CHI FOR BALANCE

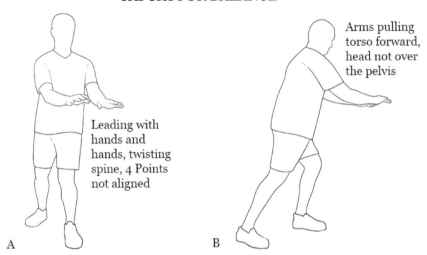

Figure 15-12: Horizontal Circles + Weight Shift + Hip Turn, common errors.

With those Basic Elements, tips, and common errors in mind, let's proceed to Exercise 25.

## Exercise 25: Horizontal Circles + Weight Shift + Hip Turn

1. **Getting Ready to Move.** Stand and settle into Neutral Posture. Take a minute, or more if you like, and stand quietly before moving.

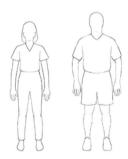

2. **Starting Position, Left Leg Forward Stance.** Shift weight back. Turn your hips into your back leg. Place your hands at the Back of your Horizontal Circle. Pick a comfortable height for your hands. (Figure 15-13A.)

3. **Make counterclockwise Horizontal Circles, 5 repetitions.** Shift weight forward, turning your hips counterclockwise into your front leg, as you extend your

### Circle #5: Horizontal Circles + Weight Shift + Hip Turn

arms, circling your hands to the Front of your Horizontal Circle. (Figure 15-13B.) Then shift weight back, turning your hips counterclockwise toward into back leg as you bend your arms, circling your hands to the Back of your Horizontal Circle. (Figure 15-13C.) After 5 repetitions, return to the Back of your Horizontal Circle.

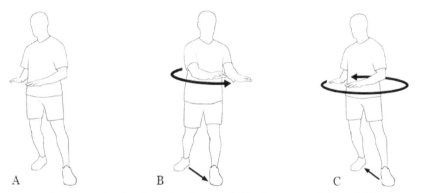

Figure 15-13: Counterclockwise Horizontal Circles + Weight Shift + Hip Turn, left leg forward.

4. **Change directions, make clockwise Horizontal Circles, 5 repetitions**. From the Back of your Horizontal Circle (Figure 15-14A), shift weight forward, turning your hips clockwise into your front leg as you extend your arms, circling your hands to the Front of your Horizontal Circle. (Figure 15-14B.) Then shift weight back, turning your hips clockwise toward your back leg, as you bend your arms, circling your hands to the Back of your Horizontal Circle. (Figure 15-14C.) After 5 repetitions, return to the Back of your Horizontal Circle.

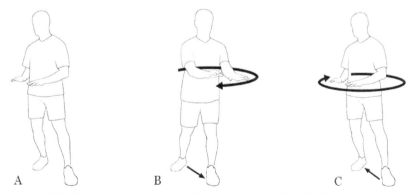

Figure 15-14: Clockwise Horizontal Circles + Weight Shift + Hip Turn, left leg forward.

5. **Change your stance to Right Leg Forward Stance**. Shift weight back. You're your hips into your back leg. Place your hands at the Back of your Horizontal Circle. (Figure 15-15A.)

6. **Make clockwise Horizontal Circles, 5 repetitions**. Shift weight forward, turning your hips clockwise into your front leg as you extend your arms, circling your hands to the Front of your Horizontal Circle. (Figure 15-15B.) Then shift weight back, turning your hips clockwise into your back leg as you bend your arms, circling your hands to the Back of your Horizontal Circle. (Figure 15-15C.) After 5 repetitions, return to the Back of your Horizontal Circle.

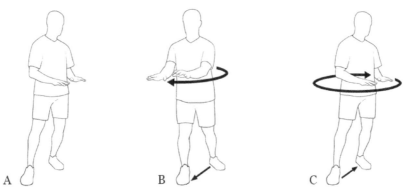

*Figure 15-15: Clockwise Horizontal Circles + Weight Shift + Hip Turn, right leg forward.*

7. **Change directions, make counterclockwise Horizontal Circles, 5 repetitions**. From the Back of your Horizontal Circle (Figure 15-6A), shift weight forward, turning your hips counterclockwise into your front leg as you extend your arms, circling your hands to the Front of your Horizontal Circle. (Figure 15-16B.) Then smoothly shift weight back, turning your hips counterclockwise into your back leg, as you bend your arms, circling the hands to the Back of your Horizontal Circle. (Figure 15-16C.) After 5 repetitions, return to the Back of your Horizontal Circle.

*Circle #5: Horizontal Circles + Weight Shift + Hip Turn*

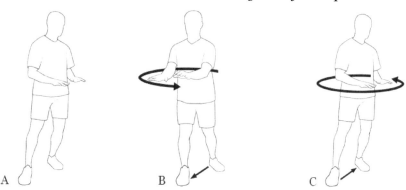

*Figure 15-16: Counterclockwise Horizontal Circles + Weight Shift + Hip Turn, right leg forward.*

8. **Conclusion**. Smoothly transition to Neutral Posture.

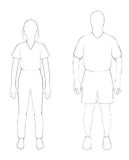

**Practice Recommendation:** Practice Exercise 25 for 1–2 days, 2-4 times each day. When you can comfortably make a set of 20 Horizontal Circles + Weight Shifts + Hip Turns, you're ready for the next exercise. It's time to add feeling your feet and center.

# Exercise 26: Horizontal Circles + Weight Shift + Hip Turn + Feeling Your Feet and Center

For the movements of Exercise 26, you can reference the instructions and figures accompanying Exercise 25.

**Practice Video.** You can also follow me in the guided practice video covering this exercise. To access the video, go to https://www.chicagotaichi.org/tai-chi-for-balance-guided-practice-videos/

1. **Getting Ready to Move.** Take a minute, or more if you like, and stand quietly before moving. First, settle into Neutral Posture. Then feel your feet, balancing the pressure in your feet. Then feel your center, aligning your center vertically. We aim to maintain a vertical center throughout the exercise.

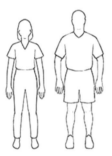 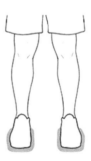 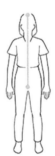

2. **Starting Position, Left Leg Forward Stance, weight back.** Turn your hips slightly into your weighted leg. Place your hands at the Back of your Horizontal Circle.

3. **Make counterclockwise Horizontal Circles, 5 repetitions.** As you move, feel your feet. Feel the constantly changing pressure in each foot. Feel your center. Maintain, or correct to, a vertical posture. After 5 repetitions, return to the Back of your Horizontal Circle.

4. **Change directions, make clockwise Horizontal Circles.** As you move, feel your feet and center as described above. After 5 repetitions, return to the Back of your Horizontal Circle.

*Circle #5: Horizontal Circles + Weight Shift + Hip Turn*

5. **Change your stance to Right Leg Forward Stance.** Shift weight back. Place your hands at the Back of your Horizontal Circle.

6. **Make clockwise Horizontal Circles + Weight Shift + Hip Turn, 5 repetitions**. As you move, feel your feet and center as described above. After 5 repetitions, return to the Back of your Horizontal Circle.

7. **Change directions, make counterclockwise Horizontal Circles + Weight Shift + Hip Turn, 5 repetitions**. As you move, feel your feet and center as described above. After 5 repetitions, return to the Back of your Horizontal Circle.

8. **Conclusion**. Smoothly transition to Neutral Posture.

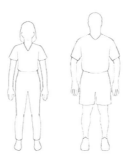

**Practice Recommendation:** Practice Exercise 26 for 1–2 days, 2–3 times each day. When you can comfortably make a set of 20 Horizontal Circles + Weight Shifts + Hip Turns while feeling your feet and center as described above, you're ready for a set of Circles #1 through #5. For that, turn to the next chapter.

# Chapter Wrap-up

This chapter introduced Circle #5: Horizontal Circles + Weight Shift + Hip Turn. Key points include:

**Make Horizontal Circles by Coordinating the Weight Shift, the Hip Turn, and the Bending and Stretching of Your Arms**

- We make Horizontal Circles mainly with the action of the legs and hips, plus the bending and stretching of the arms.
- Shifting weight back, turning your hips into your back leg, and bending your arms brings the hands to the Back of your Horizontal Circle.
- Shifting weight forward, turning your hips into your front leg, and stretching your arms sends the hands to the Front of the Horizontal Circle.
- To make counterclockwise Horizontal Circles with your hands, turn your hips counterclockwise.
- To make clockwise Horizontal Circles with your hands, turn your hips clockwise.

**Balance the Size of Your Horizontal Circle with the Size of Your Weight Shift + Hip Turn**

- We aim for connected, balanced, whole-body movement.
- If your Weight Shift + Hip Turn is smaller, balance that with a smaller Horizontal Circle.

**Continue to Hone Your Whole Body Awareness and Precise Posture Control**

- Performing Horizontal Circles + Weight Shift + Hip Turn causes constantly changing pressure in your feet. Feeling that pressure will help you stabilize an important aspect of Whole Body Awareness.
- Feeling your center and maintaining, or correcting to, a vertical posture during the movement will continue to refine your skill at Precise Posture Control.

All of this contributes to developing a more stable, fall-resistant structure through increasingly dynamic movement.

# Chapter 16

## Adding to Our Tai Chi for Balance Exercise Set: Circles #1 through #5

It's time to put Circles #1–#5 together. The increased volume of Tai Chi for Balance exercise will continue to develop strength, endurance, and flexibility in and around your legs and hips.

As your exercise volume grows, you will continue to hone Tai Chi for Balance skills, including:

- Whole Body Awareness, including feeling your feet and center.
- Increasingly Precise Posture Control, by maintaining a relaxed, upright, vertical posture, except when intentionally inclining the torso.
- Feeling and maintaining postural alignments including your knee alignments and 4 Points.

You'll achieve all of this as you move in increasingly dynamic ways.

By this point in the program, many people report how their Tai Chi for Balance skills are showing up in other parts of their life. How about for you?

For example, you may feel how you tend to lean while standing or moving. You may feel yourself adjusting automatically to a vertical posture, resulting in a more stable, more fall resistant structure.

That's Tai Chi for Balance in action!

With that, let's proceed to Exercise 27.

# Exercise 27: Circles #1 through #5

The following instructions guide you step by step through a full set of Circles #1 through #5.

**Practice Video.** You can also follow me in the guided practice video covering this exercise. To access the video, go to https://www.chicagotaichi.org/tai-chi-for-balance-guided-practice-videos/

**Getting Ready to Move**

Take a minute, or more if you like, and stand quietly before moving.

> ➤ Settle into Neutral Posture.
> ➤ Feel your feet, balancing the pressure in your feet.
> ➤ Feel your center, aligning your center vertically.

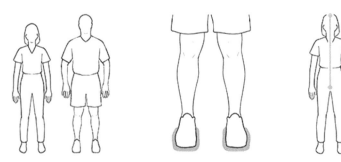

**Circle #1: Vertical Circles + Kwa Squat**

1. **Circle #1 Starting Position**. Sink into a Kwa Squat. Place your hands at the Back of your Vertical Circle. (Figure 16-1A.) Feel for any pressure changes in your feet. Feel your center inclined slightly forward.

2. **Make Top to Bottom Vertical Circles, 10 repetitions**. (Figure 16-1A-E). As you move, feel your feet and center. After each Kwa Squat, balance the pressures in your feet and return your center to the vertical. After 10 repetitions, return to the Back of your Vertical Circle.

*Adding to Our Tai Chi for Balance Exercise Set: Circles #1 through #5*

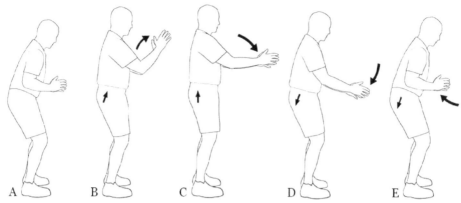

*Figure 16-1: Circle #1, Top to Bottom Vertical Circles + Kwa Squat.*

3. **Change directions; make Bottom to Top Vertical Circles.** (Figure 16-2A-E). As you move, feel your feet and center as described above. After 10 repetitions, return to the Back of your Vertical Circle. Then go to Circle #2 Starting Position.

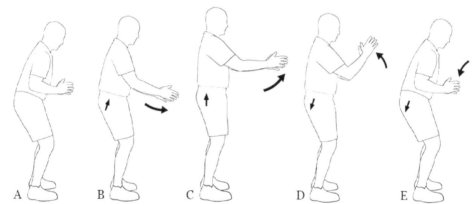

*Figure 16-2: Circle #1, Bottom to Top Vertical Circles + Kwa Squat.*

**Circle #2: Vertical Circles + Weight Shift**

1. **Starting Position, Left Leg Forward Stance.** Shift weight back. Place your hands at the Back of your Vertical Circle. (Figure 16-3A.) Feel your feet, one loaded, one unloaded. Feel your center. Establish a vertical posture.

2. **Make Top to Bottom Vertical Circles, 5 repetitions.** (Figure 16-3A-E.) As you move, feel your feet and center. Feel the constantly changing pressure in each

foot. Maintain a vertical center. After 5 repetitions, return to the Back of your Vertical Circle.

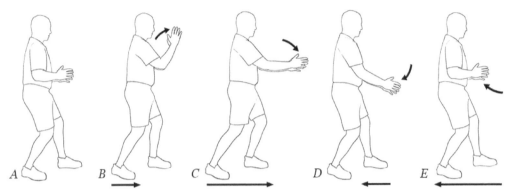

Figure 16-3: Circle #2, Top to Bottom Vertical Circles + Weight Shift, left leg forward.

3. **Change directions; make Bottom to Top Vertical Circles**. (Figure 16-4A-E.) As you move, feel your feet and center as described above. After 5 repetitions, return to the Back of your Vertical Circle.

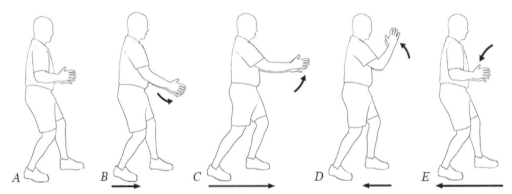

Figure 16-4: Circle 2, Bottom to Top Vertical Circles + Weight Shift, left leg forward.

4. **Change to Right Leg Forward Stance**. Shift weight back. Place your hands at the Back of your Vertical Circle. (Figure 16-5A.)

5. **Make Top to Bottom Vertical Circles, 5 repetitions**. (Figure 16-5A-E.) As you move, feel your feet and center as described above. After 5 repetitions, return to the Back of your Vertical Circle.

*Adding to Our Tai Chi for Balance Exercise Set: Circles #1 through #5*

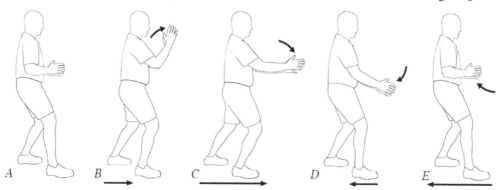

*Figure 16-5: Circle #2, Top to Bottom Vertical Circles + Weight Shift, right leg forward.*

6. **Change directions; make Bottom to Top Vertical Circles, 5 repetitions.** (Figure 16-6A-E.) As you move, feel your feet and center as described above. After 5 repetitions, return to the Back of your Vertical Circle. Then go to Circle #3 Starting Position.

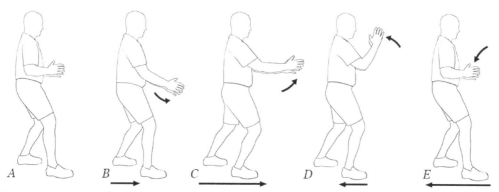

*Figure 16-6: Circle 2, Bottom to Top Vertical Circles + Weight Shift, right leg forward.*

## Circle #3: Vertical Circles + Weight Shift + Hip Turn

1. **Starting Position, Left Leg Forward Stance.** Shift weight back. Turn your hips into your back leg. Place your hands at the Back of your Vertical Circle. (Figure 16-7A.) Feel your feet, one loaded, one unloaded. Feel your center. Establish a vertical posture.

2. **Make Top to Bottom Vertical Circles + Weight Shift + Hip Turn, 5 repetitions**. (Figure 16-7A-E.) As you move, feel your feet and center. Feel the constantly changing pressure in each foot. Maintain your center in the vertical. After 5 repetitions, return to the Back of your Vertical Circle.

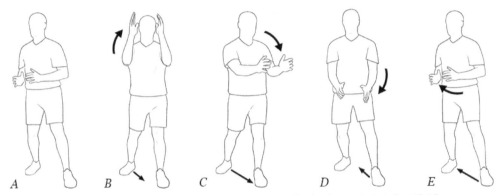

*Figure 16-7: Circle #3, Top to Bottom Vertical Circles + Weight Shift + Hip Turn, left leg forward.*

3. **Change directions; make Bottom to Top Vertical Circles**. (Figure 16-8A-E.) As you move, feel your feet and center as described above. After 5 repetitions, return to the Back of your Vertical Circle.

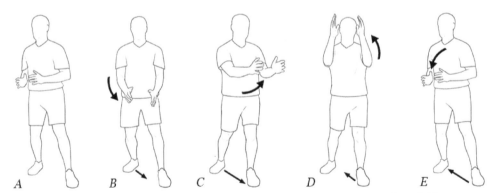

*Figure 16-8: Circle #3, Bottom to Top Vertical Circles + Weight Shift + Hip Turn, left leg forward.*

4. **Change your stance to Right Leg Forward Stance**. Shift weight back. Turn your hips into your back leg. Position your hands at the Back of your Vertical Circle. (Figure 16-9A.)

Adding to Our Tai Chi for Balance Exercise Set: Circles #1 through #5

5. **Make Top to Bottom Vertical Circles, 5 repetitions**. (Figure 16-9A-E.) As you move, feel your feet and center as described above. After 5 repetitions, return to the Back of your Vertical Circle.

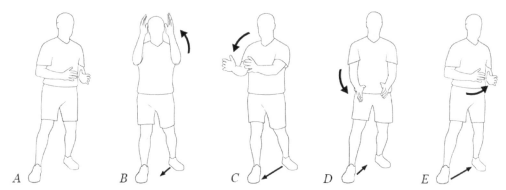

Figure 16-9: Circle #3, Top to Bottom Vertical Circles + Weight Shift + Hip Turn, right leg forward.

6. **Change directions; make Bottom to Top Vertical Circles, 5 repetitions**. (Figure 16-10A-E.) As you move, feel your feet as described above. After 5 repetitions, return to the Back of your Vertical Circle. Then proceed to Circle #4 Starting Position.

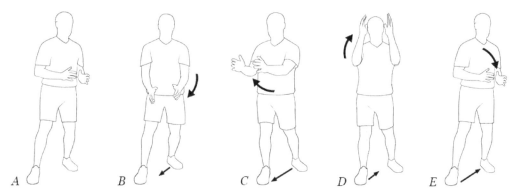

Figure 16-10: Circle #3, Bottom to Top Vertical Circles + Weight Shift + Hip Turn, right leg forward.

## Circle #4: Horizontal Circles + Kwa Squat

1. **Starting Position**. Adjust your feet to Neutral Posture position. Sink into a Kwa Squat, hips straight ahead. Place your hands at the Back of your Horizontal Circle.

Pick a comfortable height for your hands. (Figure 16-11A.) Balance the pressure in your feet. Feel your center inclined slightly forward.

2. **Make counterclockwise Horizontal Circles, 10 repetitions.** As you move, feel your feet and center. Before and after each Kwa Squat, balance the pressure in your feet and return your center to the vertical. After 10 repetitions, return to the Back of your Horizontal Circle.

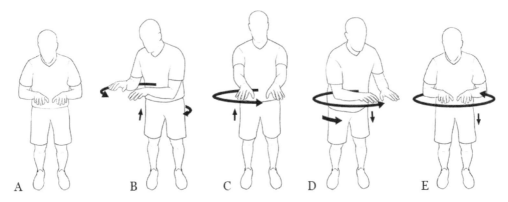

Figure 16-11: Circle #4, Counterclockwise Horizontal Circles + Kwa Squat.

3. **Change directions; make clockwise Horizontal Circles, 10 repetitions.** (Figure 16-12A-E.) As you move, feel your feet and center as described above. After 10 repetitions return to the Back of your Horizontal Circle. Then go to Circle #5 Starting Position.

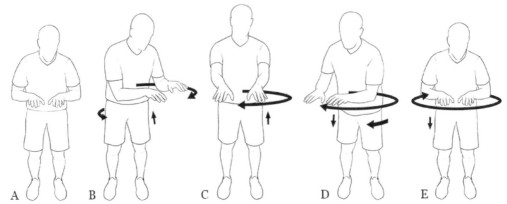

Figure 16-12: Circle #4, Clockwise Horizontal Circles + Kwa Squat.

*Adding to Our Tai Chi for Balance Exercise Set: Circles #1 through #5*

## Circle #5: Horizontal Circles + Weight Shift + Hip Turn

1. **Starting Position, Left Leg Forward Stance.** Shift weight back. Turn your hips into your back leg. Place your hands at the Back of your Horizontal Circle. (Figure 16-13A.) Feel your feet, one loaded, one unloaded. Feel your center. Establish a vertical posture.

2. **Make counterclockwise Horizontal Circles, 5 repetitions**. (Figure 16-13A-C.) As you move, feel your feet and center. Feel the constantly changing pressure in each foot. Maintain your center in the vertical. After 5 repetitions, return to the Back of your Horizontal Circle.

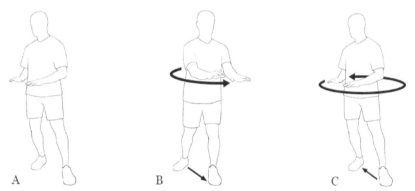

*Figure 16-13: Circle #5, Counterclockwise Horizontal Circles + Weight Shift + Hip Turn, left leg forward.*

3. **Change directions; make clockwise Horizontal Circles, 5 repetitions**. Figure 16-14A-C.) As you move, feel your feet and center as described above. After 5 repetitions, return to the Back of your Horizontal Circle.

TAI CHI FOR BALANCE

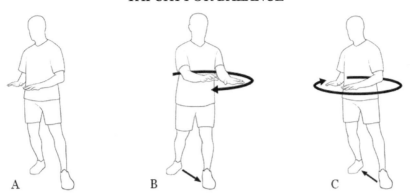

*Figure 16-14: Circle #5, Clockwise Horizontal Circles + Weight Shift + Hip Turn, left leg forward.*

4. **Change your stance to Right Leg Forward Stance.** (Figure 16-15A.) Shift weight back. Turn your hips into your back leg. Place your hands at the Back of your Horizontal Circle.

5. **Make clockwise Horizontal Circles, 5 repetitions**. (Figure 16-15A-C.) As you move, feel your feet and center as described above. After 5 repetitions, return to the Back of your Horizontal Circle.

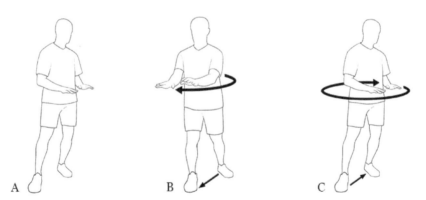

*Figure 16-15: Circle #5, Clockwise Horizontal Circles + Weight Shift + Hip Turn, right leg forward.*

6. **Change directions; make counterclockwise Horizontal Circles.** (Figure 16-16A-C.) As you move, feel your feet and center as described above. After 5 repetitions, return to the Back of your Horizontal Circle.

*Adding to Our Tai Chi for Balance Exercise Set: Circles #1 through #5*

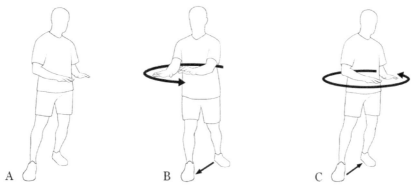

*Figure 16-16: Circle #5, Counterclockwise Horizontal Circles + Weight Shift + Hip Turn, right leg forward.*

## Conclusion

➢ **Smoothly return to Neutral Posture**.

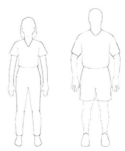

➢ **Stand in Neutral Posture for 1–2 minutes**. Notice how you feel after performing 100 Circles, 120 Weight Shifts, 40 Kwa Squats, and 80 Hip Turns.

In Exercise 27, you're performing an increasing volume of low-impact, weight-bearing exercise. This exercise will strengthen your legs and hips. Equally important, you're developing greater Whole Body Awareness and Precise Posture Control, while performing dynamic movement for longer periods. All of this combines to help you maintain an increasingly stable, fall-resistant structure.

That's what Tai Chi for Balance is all about. At this point, you are well on your way toward feeling stable, secure, and confident on your feet—and avoiding falls. Good for you!

**Practice Recommendation:** Practice Exercise 27 for 2–4 days, once each day. When you can comfortably perform a set of Circles #1–#5 while feeling your feet and center and maintaining a vertical posture (except when intentionally inclining the torso), you're ready for Part 4.

# Part 4

# Completing the Set: Coronal Circles

In Part 4, we explore the last two circles of the Tai Chi for Balance Exercise Set—**Circle #6: Coronal Circles + Kwa Squat** and **Circle #7: Coronal Circles + Weight Shift + Hip Turn**.

With Circles #6 and #7, we continue to build upon the foundation developed in Parts 1 through 3, including Whole Body Awareness, Precise Posture Control, postural alignments, knee alignments, the Kwa Squat, the Weight Shift, and the Weight Shift + Hip Turn. Upon that foundation, we change the plane of our circles to Coronal.

A "corona" is a circle surrounding a body like the sun or moon. In Circles #6 and #7, our arms and hands will move like they are going around a disc in front of us. We'll tilt the top of the disc away from us. As a result, we extend our arms and hands up and away from us at the top of the circle and bend our arms and hands down and toward us at the bottom of the circle.

Making Coronal Circles will again change the patterns of forces flowing through your body. This helps you further refine your Whole Body Awareness and Precise Posture Control. The movements also continue to strengthen and tone your hips and legs.

Separated into three short chapters, Part 4 moves quickly. By Chapter 19, you progress to 20 repetitions each of Circles #1 through #7—a full set of Tai Chi Circling Hands. By following my guidance, along with the 70% Rule and the Don't Cause Pain Rule, these exercises will help you maintain an increasingly stable, fall-resistant structure. Plus, it's wonderful low-impact exercise and fun!

Let's proceed to Chapter 17 and explore Coronal Circles.

# Chapter 17

# Circle #6:
# Coronal Circles + Kwa Squat

In this chapter, we explore Circle #6: Coronal Circles + Kwa Squat. We'll start with the Basic Elements.

## Basic Elements

1. **Starting Position**. Sink into a Kwa Squat, hips straight ahead. Place your hands in front of your lower abdomen, about one fist's distance from your body. Bend your wrists to angle the hands 15–45 degrees up from horizontal. This is the Bottom of your Coronal Circle. (Figure 17-1.)

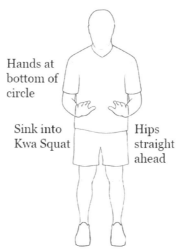

Figure 17-1: Coronal Circles + Kwa Squat, Starting Position.

2. **Make counterclockwise Coronal Circles + Kwa Squat.** We begin by making counterclockwise Coronal Circles.

3. **Right Side of Coronal Circle.** From the Bottom of your Coronal Circle, begin rising out of the Kwa Squat, turning your hips to your right, as you begin to extend and raise your arms and hands. When your arms and hands are to the right of where you started, and your hands have risen to the middle of your chest, you've reached the Right Side of your Coronal Circle. (Figure 17-2A.)

4. **Top of Coronal Circle.** Continue rising out of the Kwa Squat, turning your hips from your right to straight ahead, as you continue extending and raising your arms and hands. When you've risen fully out of your Kwa Squat, turned your hips straight ahead, and circled your hands to approximately the height of your face, you're at the Top of your Coronal Circle. (Figure 17-2B.)

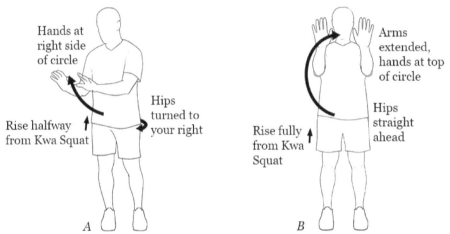

Figure 17-2: Counterclockwise Coronal Circles + Kwa Squat, Right Side and Top of Coronal Circle.

5. **Left Side of Coronal Circle.** Begin to sink into a Kwa Squat, turning your hips counterclockwise from straight ahead to your left, as you begin bending and lowering your arms and hands. When your arms and hands are to the left of where you started, and your hands have descended to a level of roughly the middle of your chest, you've reached the Left Side of your Coronal Circle. (Figure 17-3A.)

6. **Bottom of Coronal Circle.** Continue to sink into a Kwa Squat, turning your hips from your left to straight ahead, as you continue bending and lowering your arms and hands. When you've reached the bottom of your Kwa Squat, with your hips are straight ahead, and your hands at the Starting Position, you've returned to the Bottom of your Coronal Circle. (Figure 17-3B.)

## Circle #6: Coronal Circles + Kwa Squat

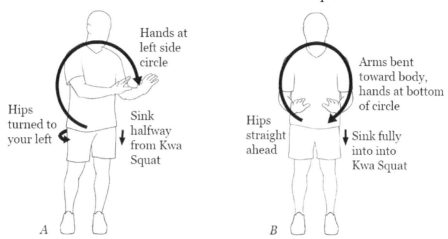

Figure 17-3: *Counterclockwise Coronal Circles + Kwa Squat, Left Side and Bottom of Coronal Circle.*

Figure 17-4 shows the movements in sequence.

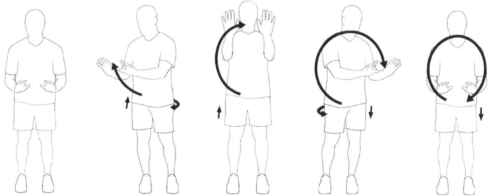

Figure 17-4: *Counterclockwise Coronal Circles + Kwa Squat.*

7. **Change directions**. Make clockwise Coronal Circles + Kwa Squat.

8. **Left Side of Coronal Circle**. From the Bottom of your Coronal Circle, begin rising out of your Kwa Squat, turning your hips to your left, as you begin extending and raising your arms and hands. When your arms and hands are to the left of where you started, and your hands have risen to about the middle of your chest, you've reached the Left Side of your Coronal Circle. (Figure 17-5A.)

253

9. **Top of Coronal Circle.** Continue to rise out of your Kwa Squat, turning your hips from your left to straight ahead, as you continue extending and raising your arms and hands. When you have risen fully out of your Kwa Squat, turned your hips straight ahead, and circled your hands to approximately the height of your face, you are at the Top of your Coronal Circle. (Figure 17-5B.)

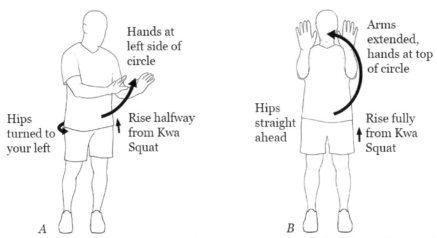

*Figure 17-5: Clockwise Coronal Circles + Kwa Squat, Left Side and Top of Coronal Circle.*

10. **Right Side of Coronal Circle.** Begin to sink into a Kwa Squat, turning your hips from straight ahead to your right, as you begin bending and lowering your arms and hands. When your arms and hands are to the right of where you started, and your hands have descended to a level of roughly the middle of your chest, you've reached the Right Side of your Coronal Circle. (Figure 17-6A.)

11. **Bottom of Coronal Circle.** Continue to sink into a Kwa Squat, turning your hips from your right to straight ahead, as you continue bending and lowering your arms and hands. When you've reached the bottom of your Kwa Squat, with your hips straight ahead, and your hands at the Starting Position, you've returned to the Bottom of your Coronal Circle. (Figure 17-6B.)

## Circle #6: Coronal Circles + Kwa Squat

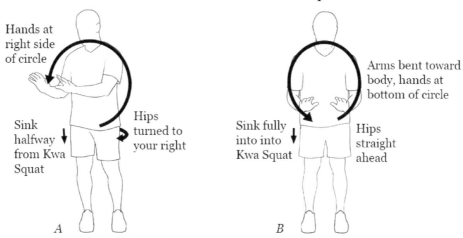

Figure 17-6: Clockwise Coronal Circles + Kwa Squat, Right Side and Bottom of Coronal Circle.

Figure 17-7 shows the movements in sequence.

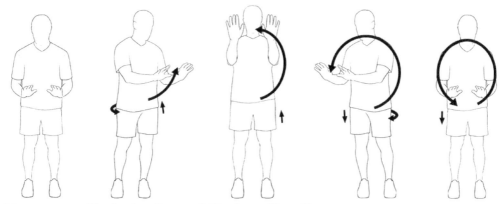

Figure 17-7: Clockwise Coronal Circles + Kwa Squat.

As you begin to practice Coronal Circles + Kwa Squat, I recommend you review the *Tips and Common Errors* in the next section. From your experience in performing Vertical and Horizontal Circles, these pointers will sound familiar.

## Tips and Common Errors

*Tips*

**Make Coronal Circles by turning the hips slightly as you perform Kwa Squats, plus stretching/raising the arms and bending/lowering the arms.** To make the arms and hands circle counterclockwise, turn your hips counterclockwise. To make your arms and hands circle clockwise, rotate your hips clockwise.

To move your arms and hands up and away from the body, rise out of your Kwa Squat, as you extend and raise your arms. To move your arms and hands down and toward the body, sink into a Kwa Squat, as you bend and lower your arms.

When you combine these movement components, your hands will make Coronal Circles. The arms and hands generally stay oriented in front of the torso, extending to reach the Top of the Coronal Circle, and bending to return to the Bottom of the Coronal Circle.

**Balance the movements of the upper body with the movements of the lower body.** Aim for balance between your arm movements and your waist and leg movements. Put another way, if your Kwa Squat is small (it's okay if it is), keep your Coronal Circle small. This will help you move in a more connected manner, powering and controlling your arms with your legs and waist.

**Feel the stretch and release in your back, shoulders, and neck.** As you perform the movements, feel your back, shoulders, and neck. As the arms extend and rise, you'll feel a light stretch in those areas. As the arms bend and descend, you'll feel a release. With practice, the sensations of stretching and releasing become smooth and continuous.

*Common Errors*

**Making Coronal Circles by twisting the spine.** A common error is to circle to the Left Side or Right Side of the Coronal Circle with the arms and shoulders rather than rotating the hips. This twists the spine and breaks the alignment of the 4 Points. (Figure 17-8A.)

*Circle #6: Coronal Circles + Kwa Squat*

**Locking the elbows at the Top of the Coronal Circle.** A common error when moving the hands toward the Top of the Coronal Circle is to lock the elbows. This creates tension and tightness in the arms and shoulders. (Figure 17-8B.)

**Tensing the hands and fingers.** A common error is tensing the hands and fingers, especially as you stretch toward the Top of the Coronal Circle. This makes the hands and fingers stiff and can contribute to tension in other parts of the body. (Figure 17-8C.)

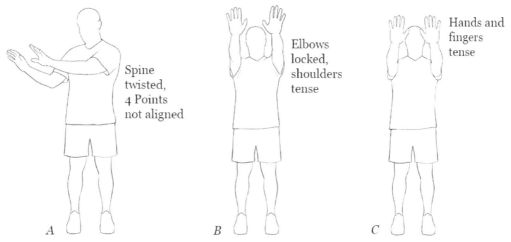

Figure 17-8: *Coronal Circles + Kwa Squat, common errors.*

With those Basic Elements, tips, and common errors in mind, let's proceed to Exercise 28.

TAI CHI FOR BALANCE

# Exercise 28: Coronal Circles + Kwa Squat

1. **Getting Ready to Move.** Stand and settle into Neutral Posture. Take a minute, or more if you like, and stand quietly before moving.

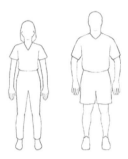

2. **Starting Position.** Sink into a Kwa Squat, hips straight ahead. Place your hands at the Bottom of your Coronal Circle. (Figure 17-9A.)

3. **Make counterclockwise Coronal Circles, 10 repetitions.** From the Starting Position, rise from your Kwa Squat, turning your hips to your right then straight ahead, as you extend and raise your arms, circling your hands counterclockwise through the Right Side and Top of your Coronal Circle. (Figure 17-9B-C.) Then sink into a Kwa Squat, turning your hips to your left then straight ahead, as you bend and lower your arms, circling your hands counterclockwise through the Left Side and Bottom of your Coronal Circle. (Figure 17-9D-E.) After 10 repetitions, return to the Bottom of your Coronal Circle. (Figure 17-10A.)

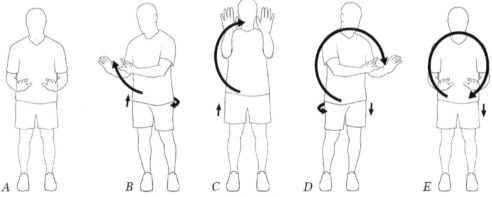

*Figure 17-9: Counterclockwise Coronal Circles + Kwa Squat.*

*Circle #6: Coronal Circles + Kwa Squat*

4. **Change directions; make clockwise Coronal Circles, 10 repetitions**. Rise from your Kwa Squat, turning your hips to your left then straight ahead, as you extend and raise your arms, circling your hands clockwise through the Left Side and Top of your Coronal Circle. (Figure 17-10B-C.) Then sink into a Kwa Squat, turning your hips to your right then straight ahead, as you bend and lower your arms, circling your hands clockwise through the Right Side and Bottom of your Coronal Circle. (Figure 17-10D-E.) After 10 repetitions, return to the Bottom of your Coronal Circle.

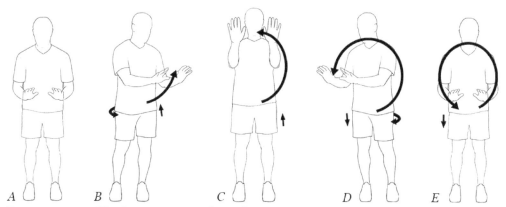

*Figure 17-10: Clockwise Coronal Circles + Kwa Squat.*

5. **Conclusion**. Smoothly transition to Neutral Posture.

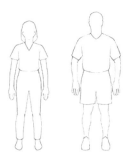

**Practice Recommendation:** Practice Exercise 28 for 1–2 days, 2–4 times each day. When you can comfortably make a set of 20 Coronal Circles + Kwa Squats, you're ready for the next exercise. It's time to add feeling your feet and center.

TAI CHI FOR BALANCE

# Exercise 29: Coronal Circles + Kwa Squat + Feeling Your Feet and Center

For the movements of Exercise 29, you can reference the instructions and figures accompanying Exercise 28.

**Practice Video.** You can also follow me in the guided practice video covering this exercise. To access the video, go to https://www.chicagotaichi.org/tai-chi-for-balance-guided-practice-videos/

1. **Getting Ready to Move.** Take a minute, or more if you like, and stand quietly before moving. First, settle into Neutral Posture. Then feel your feet, balancing the pressure in your feet. Then feel your center, aligning your center vertically.

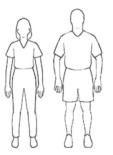 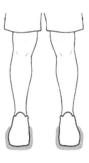 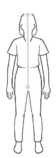

2. **Starting Position**. Sink into a Kwa Squat, hips straight ahead. Place your hands at the Bottom of your Coronal Circle.

3. **Make counterclockwise Coronal Circles, 10 repetitions**. As you move, feel your feet and center. Before and after each Kwa Squat, balance the pressures in your feet and return your center to the vertical. After 10 repetitions, return to the Back of your Vertical Circle.

4. **Change directions; make clockwise Coronal Circles, 10 repetitions.** As you move, feel your feet and center as described above. After 10 repetitions, return to the Bottom of your Coronal Circle.

5. **Conclusion**. Smoothly transition to Neutral Posture.

*Circle #6: Coronal Circles + Kwa Squat*

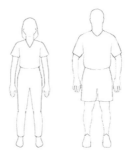

**Practice Recommendation:** Practice Exercise 29 1–2 days, 2–3 times each day. When you can comfortably make a set of 20 Coronal Circles + Kwa Squats, while feeling your feet and center as described above, you're ready for the next chapter.

It's time to add the Weight Shift + Hip Turn to our Coronal Circles.

# Chapter Wrap-up

This chapter introduced Circle #6: Coronal Circles + Kwa Squat. Key points include:

**Making Coronal Circles + Kwa Squat**

- Coronal Circles are like tracing the face of an analog clock in front of you, with the top of the clock face tilted away from you.
- Coronal Circles + Kwa Squat have a Bottom, Top, Right Side, and Left Side.
- You want to develop a sense of making Coronal Circles mainly with the action of your legs and hips, plus bending/lowering and stretching/raising your arms.
- To make counterclockwise Coronal Circles with your hands, rotate your hips counterclockwise. To make clockwise Coronal Circles with your hands, rotate your hips clockwise.
- Sinking into the Kwa Squat plus bending/lowering the arms brings the hands to the Bottom of your Coronal Circle.
- Rising from the Kwa Squat plus stretching/raising the arms sends the hands to the Top of the Coronal Circle.

**Balance the Size of Your Coronal Circle with the Size of your Kwa Squat.**

- We're aiming for connected, balanced, whole-body movement.
- If your Kwa Squat is smaller, balance that with a smaller Coronal Circle.

**Honing Your Whole Body Awareness and Precise Posture Control**

- Performing Coronal Circles + Kwa Squat will result in different patterns of force through your body.
- Feeling your feet and balancing the pressures in your feet, combined with feeling your center and maintaining a vertical posture (except when intentionally inclining the torso in a Kwa Squat) will continue to train your Whole Body Awareness and Precise Posture Control.

# Chapter 18

# Circle #7:
# Coronal Circles + Weight Shift + Hip Turn

For our last circle, Circle #7, we add the Weight Shift + Hip Turn to our Coronal Circles, putting more leg and hip action into the movements. Practicing Circle #7 will:

- ➢ Strengthen, stretch, and improve circulation in the entire lower half of the body.
- ➢ Stretch, release tension, and improve circulation in the entire upper half of the body.
- ➢ Train the nervous system to coordinate smooth, connected, whole-body movement, powering and controlling the top half of the body from the bottom half of the body.

Compared to Vertical Circles and Horizontal Circles, Coronal Circles introduce different patterns of force through the body. As part of the Tai Chi for Balance System, Circle #7 helps you to further sharpen your Whole Body Awareness and Precise Posture Control. In doing so, you'll increasingly maintain a stable, fall-resistant structure.

Let's begin with the Basic Elements of Circle #7.

## Basic Elements

1. **Starting Position, Left Leg Forward Stance**. Shift weight back. Turn your hips into your back leg. Place your hands at the Bottom of your Coronal Circle, roughly in front of your lower abdomen, about one fist's distance from your body, bending your wrists to angle the hands 15–45 degrees up from horizontal. (Figure 18-1.) We start by making counterclockwise Coronal Circles.

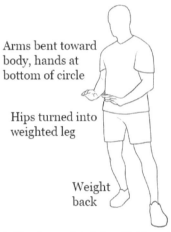

*Figure 18-1: Coronal Circles + Weight Shift + Hip Turn, left leg forward, Starting Position.*

2. **Top of Coronal Circle**. From the Starting Position, shift weight forward, turning your hips counterclockwise toward your front leg as you extend and raise your arms, circling your hands counterclockwise to the Top of your Coronal Circle. (Figure 18-2A.) Coordinate your movements so you complete the Weight Shift + Hip Turn as your hands reach the Top of your Coronal Circle.

3. **Bottom of Coronal Circle.** Shift weight back, turning your hips counterclockwise until turned into your back leg, as you bend and lower your arms, circling your hands counterclockwise to return to the Bottom of your Coronal Circle. (Figure 18-2B.) Coordinate your movements so you complete the Weight Shift + Hip Turn as your hands reach the Bottom of your Coronal Circle.

## Circle #7: Coronal Circles + Weight Shift + Hip Turn

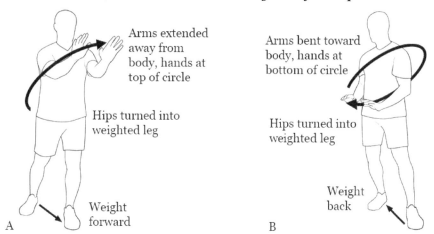

Figure 18-2: *Counterclockwise Coronal Circles + Weight Shift + Hip Turn, left leg forward, Top and Bottom of Coronal Circle.*

Figure 18-3 shows two repetitions of this movement.

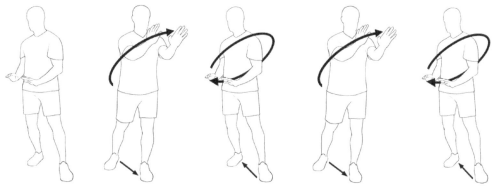

Figure 18-3: *Counterclockwise Coronal Circles + Weight Shift + Hip Turn, left leg forward.*

4. **Change directions**. From the Bottom of your Coronal Circle (Figure 18-4), change the direction of your Coronal Circles to clockwise.

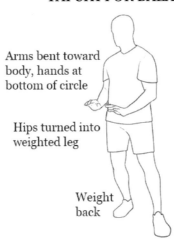

*Figure 18-4: Clockwise Coronal Circles + Weight Shift + Hip Turn, left leg forward, Bottom of Circle.*

5. **Top of Coronal Circle**. Shift weight forward, turning your hips clockwise until turned into your front leg as you extend and raise your arms, circling your hands clockwise to reach the Top of your Coronal Circle. (Figure 18-5A.) Coordinate your movements so you complete the Weight Shift + Hip Turn as your hands reach the Top of the Coronal Circle.

6. **Bottom of Coronal Circle.** Shift weight back, turning your hips clockwise until turned into your back leg as you bend and your lower arms, circling your hands clockwise to return to the Bottom of your Coronal Circle. (Figure 18-5B.) Coordinate your movements so you complete the Weight Shift + Hip Turn as your hands reach the Bottom of the Coronal Circle.

## Circle #7: Coronal Circles + Weight Shift + Hip Turn

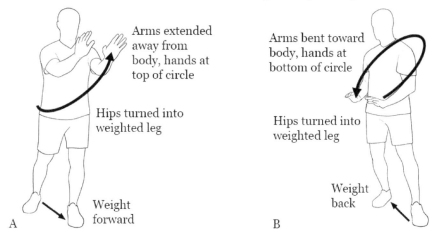

Figure 18-5: Clockwise Coronal Circles + Weight Shift + Hip Turn, left leg forward, Top and Bottom of Coronal Circle.

Figure 18-6 shows two repetitions of this movement.

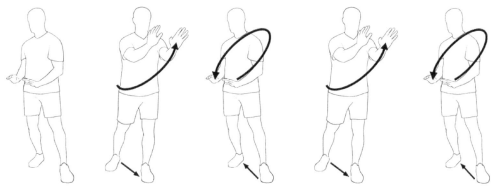

Figure 18-6: Clockwise Coronal Circles + Weight Shift + Hip Turn, left leg forward.

7. **Change your stance to Right Leg Forward Stance**. Shift your weight back. Turn your hips into your weighted leg. Position your hands at the Bottom of your Coronal Circle. (Figure 18-7.) With the right leg forward, we start with clockwise Coronal Circles.

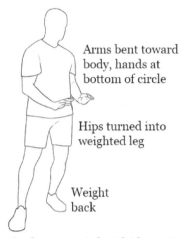

*Figure 18-7: Clockwise Coronal Circles + Weight Shift + Hip Turn, right leg forward, Bottom of Circle.*

8. **Top of Coronal Circle**. Shift weight forward, turning your hips clockwise until turned into your front leg as you extend and raise your arms, circling your hands clockwise to reach the Top of your Coronal Circle. (Figure 18-8A.) Coordinate your movements so you complete the Weight Shift + Hip Turn as your hands reach the Top of the Coronal Circle.

9. **Bottom of Coronal Circle.** Shift weight back, turning your hips clockwise until turned into your back leg as you bend and lower your arms, circling your hands clockwise to return to the Bottom of your Coronal Circle. (Figure 18-8B.) Coordinate your movements so you complete the Weight Shift + Hip Turn as your hands reach the Bottom of the Coronal Circle.

## Circle #7: Coronal Circles + Weight Shift + Hip Turn

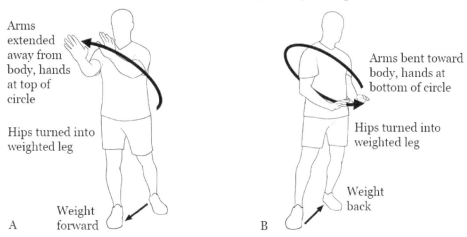

Figure 18-8: Clockwise Coronal Circles + Weight Shift + Hip Turn, right leg forward, Top and Bottom of Coronal Circle.

Figure 18-9 shows two repetitions of this movement.

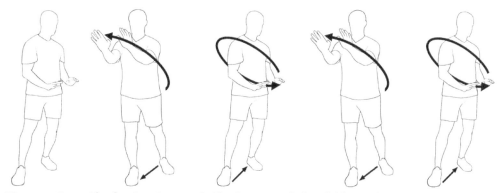

Figure 18-9: Clockwise Coronal Circles + Weight Shift + Hip Turn, right leg forward.

10. **Change directions**. Starting from the Bottom of your Coronal Circle (Figure 18-10), change the direction of your Coronal Circles to counterclockwise.

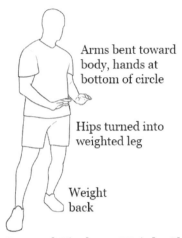

*Figure 18-10: Counterclockwise Coronal Circles + Weight Shift + Hip Turn, right leg forward, Bottom of Circle.*

11. **Top of Coronal Circle.** Shift weight forward, turning your hips counterclockwise until turned into your front leg as you extend and raise your arms, circling your hands counterclockwise to reach the Top of your Coronal Circle. (Figure 18-11A.) Coordinate your movements so you complete the Weight Shift + Hip Turn as your hands reach the Top of your Coronal Circle.

12. **Bottom of Coronal Circle.** Shift weight back, turning your hips counterclockwise until turned into your back leg as you bend and your lower arms, circling your hands counterclockwise to return to the Bottom of your Coronal Circle. (Figure 18-11B.) Coordinate your movements so you complete the Weight Shift + Hip Turn as your hands reach the Bottom of your Coronal Circle.

## Circle #7: Coronal Circles + Weight Shift + Hip Turn

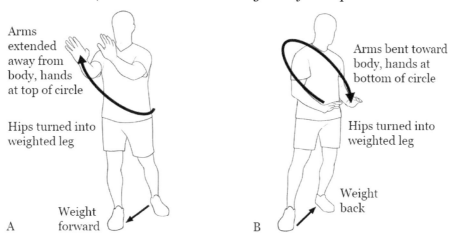

Figure 18-11: *Counterclockwise Coronal Circles + Weight Shift + Hip Turn, right leg forward, Top and Bottom of Coronal Circle.*

Figure 18-12 shows two repetitions of the movement.

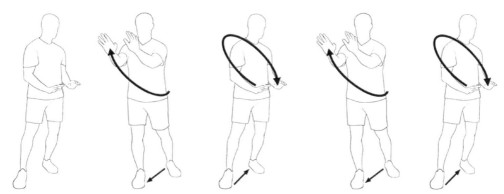

Figure 18-12: *Counterclockwise Coronal Circles + Weight Shift + Hip Turn, right leg forward.*

As you begin to practice Circle #7, I encourage you to review the following *Tips and Common Errors*. With your experience from Circles #1–#6, these pointers will sound familiar.

## Tips and Common Errors

*Tips*

**Make Coronal Circles by shifting weight, turning the hips, plus stretching/raising the arms and bending/lowering the arms.** To move the arms and hands up and away from the body, shift your weight forward, turning your hips into your front leg while extending and raising the arms. To bring the arms and hands back toward the body, shift your weight back, turning your hips into your back leg while bending and lowering the arms. The arms and hands stay oriented in front of the torso, pointing in the same direction as the front of the hips.

**Balance the size of your Coronal Circle with the size of your Weight Shift + Hip Turn.** If your Weight Shift + Hip Turn are small, your Coronal Circles will be smaller. That's fine. You are aiming for connected, balanced, whole-body movement.

*Common Errors*

**Leading with the shoulders, arms, and hands.** When adding rotation, a common error is leading the rotation with the shoulders, arms, and hands, especially when moving toward the Top of the Coronal Circle. This misaligns the 4 Points, twists the spine, and disconnects the top half of the body from the lower half of the body. (Figure 18-13A.)

**Allowing the arms to pull the torso forward.** When shifting weight forward and circling the arms up and forward, a common error is to allow the arms to pull the torso forward, resulting in a forward lean at the Top of the Coronal Circle. (Figure 18-13B.)

*Circle #7: Coronal Circles + Weight Shift + Hip Turn*

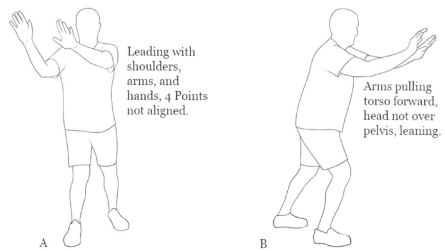

Figure 18-13: *Coronal Circles + Weight Shift + Hip Turn, common errors.*

With those Basic Elements, tips, and common errors in mind, let's proceed to Exercise 30.

## Exercise 30: Coronal Circles + Weight Shift + Hip Turn

1. **Getting Ready to Move.** Stand and settle into Neutral Posture. Take a minute, or more if you like, and stand quietly before moving.

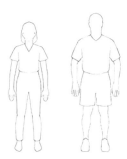

2. **Starting Position, Left Leg Forward Stance.** Shift weight back. Turn your hips into your weighted leg. Place your hands at the Bottom of your Coronal Circle. (Figure 18-14A.)

3. **Make counterclockwise Coronal Circles + Hip Turn, 5 repetitions.** From the Starting Position, smoothly shift weight forward, turning your hips

counterclockwise until turned into your front leg as you extend and raise your arms to the Top of your Coronal Circle. (Figure 18-14B.) Then smoothly shift weight back, turning your hips counterclockwise until turned into your back leg as you bend and lower your arms to the Bottom of your Coronal Circle. (Figure 18-14C.) After 5 repetitions, return to the Bottom of your Coronal Circle.

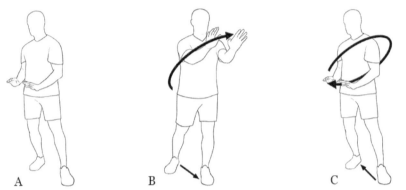

*Figure 18-14: Counterclockwise Coronal Circles + Weight Shift + Hip Turn, left leg forward.*

4. **Change directions; make clockwise Coronal Circles, 5 repetitions.** From the Bottom of your Coronal Circle (Figure 18-15A), smoothly shift weight forward, turning your hips clockwise until they're turned into your front leg as you extend and raise your arms to the Top of your Coronal Circle. (Figure 18-15B.) Then smoothly shift weight back, turning your hips clockwise until turned into your back leg as you bend and lower your arms to the Bottom of your Coronal Circle. (Figure 18-15C.) After 5 repetitions, return to the Bottom of your Coronal Circle.

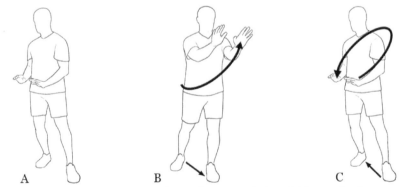

*Figure 18-15: Clockwise Coronal Circles + Weight Shift + Hip Turn, left leg forward.*

*Circle #7: Coronal Circles + Weight Shift + Hip Turn*

5. **Change your stance to Right Leg Forward Stance.** Shift weight back. Turn your hips slightly into your weighted leg. Place your hands at the Bottom of your Coronal Circle. (Figure 18-16A.)

6. **Make clockwise Coronal Circles, 5 repetitions.** From the Bottom of your Coronal Circle, smoothly shift weight forward, turning your hips clockwise until turned into your front leg as you extend and raise your arms to the Top of your Coronal Circle. (Figure 18-16B.) Then smoothly shift weight back, turning your hips clockwise until turned into your back leg as you bend and lower your arms to the Bottom of your Coronal Circle. (Figure 18-16C.) After 5 repetitions, return to the Bottom of your Coronal Circle.

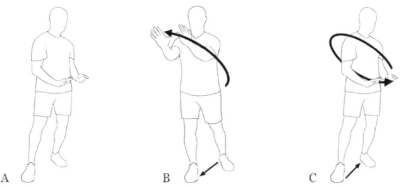

*Figure 18-16: Clockwise Coronal Circles + Weight Shift + Hip Turn, right leg forward.*

7. **Change directions; make counterclockwise Coronal Circles, 5 repetitions.** From the Bottom of your Coronal Circle (Figure 18-17A), shift weight forward, turning your hips counterclockwise until turned into your front leg as you extend and raise your arms to the Top of your Coronal Circle. (Figure 18-17B.) Then, smoothly shift weight back, turning your hips counterclockwise until turned into your back leg as you bend and lower your arms to the Bottom of your Coronal Circle. (Figure 18-17C.) After 5 repetitions, return to the Bottom of your Coronal Circle.

TAI CHI FOR BALANCE

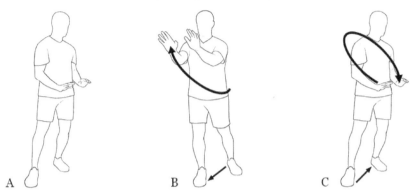

A    B    C

*Figure 18-17: Counterclockwise Coronal Circles + Weight Shift + Hip Turn, right leg forward.*

8. **Conclusion**. Smoothly transition to Neutral Posture.

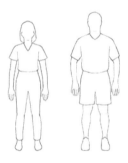

**Practice Recommendation:** Practice Exercise 30 for 1–2 days, 2–3 times each day. When you can comfortably make a set of 20 Coronal Circles + Weight Shifts + Hip Turns, you're ready for the next exercise. It's time to add feeling your feet and center.

*Circle #7: Coronal Circles + Weight Shift + Hip Turn*

# Exercise 31: Coronal Circles + Weight Shift + Hip Turn + Feeling Your Feet and Center

For the movements of Exercise 31, you can reference the instructions and figures accompanying Exercise 30.

**Practice Video.** You can also follow me in the guided practice video covering this exercise. To access the video, go to https://www.chicagotaichi.org/tai-chi-for-balance-guided-practice-videos/

1. **Getting Ready to Move.** Take a minute, or more if you like, and stand quietly before moving. First, settle into Neutral Posture. Then feel your feet, balancing the pressure in your feet. Then feel your center, establishing a vertical posture.

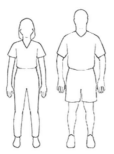 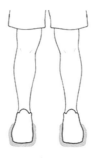 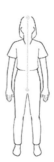

2. **Starting Position, Left Leg Forward Stance, weight back.** Turn your hips into your weighted leg. Place your hands at the Bottom of your Coronal Circle.

3. **Make counterclockwise Coronal Circles, 5 repetitions**. As you move, feel your feet. Feel the constantly changing pressure in each foot. Feel your center. Maintain, or correct to, a vertical posture. After 5 repetitions, return to the Bottom of your Coronal Circle.

4. **Change directions; make clockwise Horizontal Circles.** As you move, feel your feet and center as described above. After 5 repetitions, return to the Bottom of your Coronal Circle.

5. **Change your stance to Right Leg Forward Stance**. Shift weight back. Turn your hips into your weighted leg. Place your hands at the Bottom of your Coronal Circle.

6. **Make clockwise Coronal Circles, 5 repetitions**. As you move, feel your feet and center as described above. After 5 repetitions, return to the Bottom of your Coronal Circle.

7. **Change directions; make counterclockwise Horizontal Circles, 5 repetitions.** As you move, feel your feet and center as described above. After 5 repetitions, return to the Bottom of your Coronal Circle.

8. **Conclusion**. Smoothly transition to Neutral Posture.

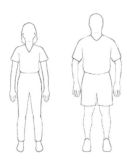

**Practice Recommendation:** Practice Exercise 31 for 1–2 days, 2–3 times each day. When you can comfortably make a set of 20 Coronal Circles + Weight Shifts + Hip Turns— while feeling your feet and center as described above, you're ready for the next chapter.

It's time for a full set of Circles #1 through #7!

*Circle #7: Coronal Circles + Weight Shift + Hip Turn*

# Chapter Wrap-up

This chapter introduced Circle #7: Coronal Circles + Weight Shift + Hip Turn. Here's a summary of key points.

**Make Coronal Circles by Coordinating the Weight Shift, the Hip Turn, Stretching/Raising the arms, and Bending/Lowering the Arms**

- You want to make Coronal Circles mainly with the action of the legs and hips, combined with stretching/raising the arms and bending/lowering the arms.
- Shifting weight back, turning your hips into your back leg, plus bending and lowering your arms, brings your hands to the Bottom of the Coronal Circle.
- Shifting weight forward, turning your hips into your front leg, plus stretching and raising your arms, sends your hands to the Top of the Coronal Circle.

**Balance the Size of Your Coronal Circle with the Size of your Weight Shift + Hip Turn**

- We're aiming for connected, balanced, whole-body movement.
- If your Weight Shift + Hip Turn is smaller, balance that with a smaller Coronal Circle.

**Honing Your Whole Body Awareness and Precise Posture Control**

- Performing Coronal Circles + Weight Shift + Hip Turn causes constantly changing pressures in your feet. Feeling those pressures and balancing them on each foot will help you maintain increasingly consistent awareness of your feet, a key element of Whole Body Awareness.
- Maintaining, or correcting to, a vertical posture during the movement will increase your sensitivity to feeling your center, refining your skill at Precise Posture Control.

All of this contributes to developing a more stable, fall-resistant structure through increasingly dynamic movement.

# Chapter 19

# Putting It All Together: Circles #1 through #7

This chapter leads you through a full set of Tai Chi Circling Hands. A full set consists of 20 repetitions each of Circles #1–#7, a total of 140 movements. That's a high volume of low-impact exercise.

More importantly, when combined with Whole Body Awareness and Precise Posture Control, the exercise trains you to maintain an increasingly strong, stable, fall-resistant structure through increasingly dynamic movement.

That's Tai Chi for Balance in action!

## Circles #1 through #7: Applying Key Principles

Throughout the set, we aim to incorporate the following Tai Chi for Balance principles:

- **The 70% Rule.** Perform each movement within a range of motion that's no more than 70% of your maximum. This allows your joints to stay soft, not locked, and your muscles and other soft tissue to remain relaxed.
- **The Don't Cause Pain Rule.** If any movement causes pain, the point of pain becomes your 100%. Back off from there until you move in a pain-free range of motion, regardless of how small that range of motion is.
- **Maintaining alignments.** Your alignments include: 1) tailbone relaxed down, 2) midriff open, 3) occiput lifted, 4) top of the head aligned vertically over the bottom of the pelvis, 5) each knee over the foot, kneecap aligned with toes, and 6) your 4 Points aligned.
- **Whole Body Awareness.** As you move, aim to maintain awareness of as much of your body as you can. Feeling your feet and center will help.
- **Precise Posture Control.** As you move, aim to maintain a vertical posture, except when intentionally inclining the torso in a Kwa Squat.

By following the step-by-step Tai Chi for Balance System, you've had plenty of practice applying these principles. Keep it up!

With that, let's proceed to a full set of Tai Chi Circling Hands. The following instructions guide you through the full set.

**Practice Video.** You can also follow me in the guided practice video covering this exercise. To access the video, go to https://www.chicagotaichi.org/tai-chi-for-balance-guided-practice-videos/

# Exercise 32: Circles #1 through #7

**Getting Ready to Move**

Take a minute, or more if you like, and stand quietly before moving.

- ➢ Settle into Neutral Posture.
- ➢ Feel your feet, balancing the pressure in your feet.
- ➢ Feel your center, aligning your center vertically.

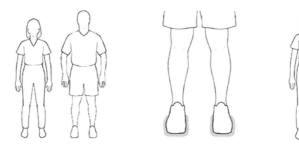

**Circle #1: Vertical Circles + Kwa Squat**

1. **Circle #1 Starting Position**. Sink into a Kwa Squat. Place your hands at the Back of your Vertical Circle. (Figure 19-1A.)

2. **Make Top to Bottom Vertical Circles, 10 repetitions**. (Figure 19-1A-E.) As you move, feel your feet and center. Before and after each Kwa Squat, balance the pressures in your feet and return your center to the vertical. After 10 repetitions, return to the Back of your Vertical Circle.

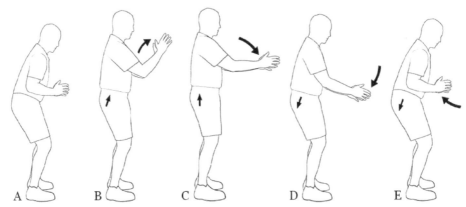

*Figure 19-1: Circle #1, Top to Bottom Vertical Circles + Kwa Squat.*

3. **Change directions; make Bottom to Top Vertical Circles**. (Figure 19-2A-E). As you move, feel your feet and center as described above. After 10 repetitions, return to the Back of your Vertical Circle. Then go to Circle #2 Starting Position.

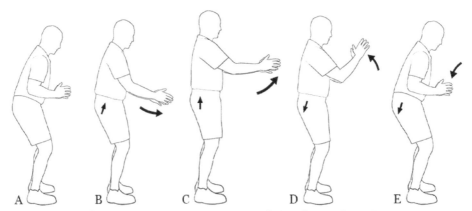

*Figure 19-2: Circle #1, Bottom to Top Vertical Circles + Kwa Squat.*

**Circle #2: Vertical Circles + Weight Shift**

1. **Starting Position, Left Leg Forward Stance**. Shift weight back. Place your hands at the Back of your Vertical Circle. (Figure 19-3A.)

2. **Make Top to Bottom Vertical Circles, 5 repetitions**. (Figure 19-3A-E.) As you move, feel your feet. Feel the constantly changing pressure in each foot. Feel your center. Maintain, or correct to, a vertical posture. After 5 repetitions, return to the Back of your Vertical Circle.

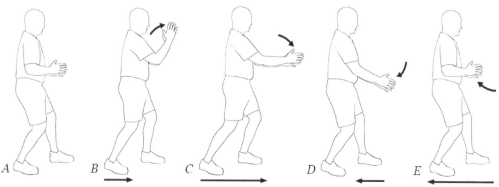

*Figure 19-3: Circle #2, Top to Bottom Vertical Circles + Weight Shift, left leg forward.*

3. **Change directions; make Bottom to Top Vertical Circles, 5 repetitions.** (Figure 19-4A-E). As you move, feel your feet and center as described above. After 5 repetitions, return to the Back of your Vertical Circle.

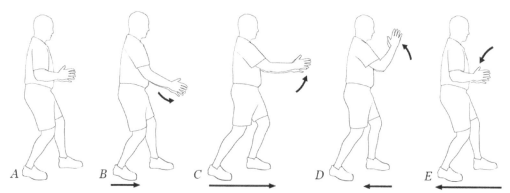

*Figure 19-4: Circle #2, Bottom to Top Vertical Circles + Weight Shift, left leg forward.*

4. **Change your stance to Right Leg Forward Stance.** Shift weight back. (Figure 19-5A.)

5. **Make Top to Bottom Vertical Circles, 5 repetitions.** (Figure 19-5A-E.) As you move, feel your feet and center as described above. After 5 repetitions, return to the Back of your Vertical Circle.

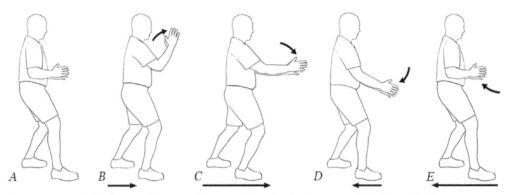

*Figure 19-5: Circle #2, Top to Bottom Vertical Circles + Weight Shift, right leg forward.*

6. **Change directions; make Bottom to Top Vertical Circles.** (Figure 19-6A-E.) As you move, feel your feet and center as described above. After 5 repetitions, return to the Back of your Vertical Circle. Then go to Circle #3 Starting Position.

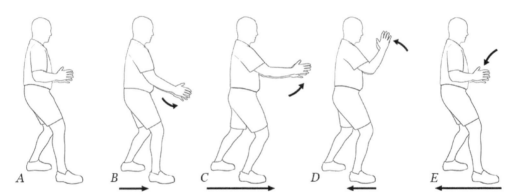

*Figure 19-6: Circle #2, Bottom to Top Vertical Circles + Weight Shift, right leg forward.*

**Circle #3: Vertical Circles + Weight Shift + Hip Turn**

1. **Starting Position, Left Leg Forward Stance.** Shift weight back. Turn your hips into your weighted leg. Place your hands at the Back of your Vertical Circle. (Figure 19-7A.)

2. **Make Top to Bottom Vertical Circles, 5 repetitions.** (Figure 19-7A-E.) As you move, feel your feet. Feel the constantly changing pressure in each foot. Feel

*Putting It All Together: Circles #1 through #7*

your center. Maintain, or correct to, a vertical posture. After 5 repetitions, return to the Back of your Vertical Circle.

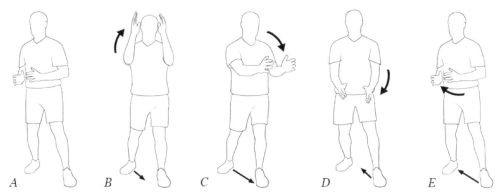

*Figure 19-7: Circle #3, Top to Bottom Vertical Circles + Weight Shift + Hip Turn, left leg forward.*

3. **Change directions; make Bottom to Top Vertical Circles, 5 repetitions**. (Figure 19-8A-E.) As you move, feel your feet and center as described above. After 5 repetitions, return to the Back of your Vertical Circle.

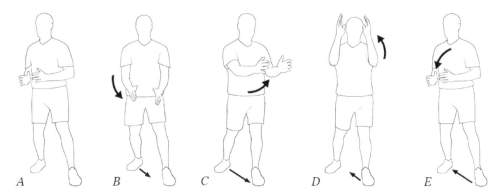

*Figure 19-8: Circle #3, Bottom to Top Vertical Circles + Weight Shift + Hip Turn, left leg forward.*

4. **Change your stance to Right Leg Forward Stance**. Shift weight back. Turn your hips into your weighted leg. (Figure 19-9A.)

5. **Make Top to Bottom Vertical Circles, 5 repetitions**. (Figure 19-9A-E.) As you move, feel your feet and center as described above. After 5 repetitions, return to the Back of your Vertical Circle.

TAI CHI FOR BALANCE

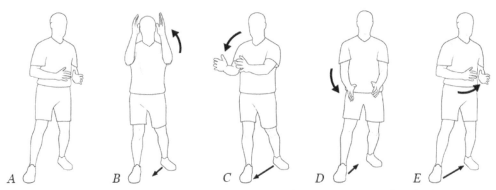

A  B  C  D  E

*Figure 19-9: Circle #3, Top to Bottom Vertical Circles + Weight Shift + Hip Turn, right leg forward.*

6. **Change directions; make Bottom to Top Vertical Circles**. (Figure 19-10a-E.) As you move, feel your feet and center as described above. After 5 repetitions, return to the Back of your Vertical Circle. Proceed to Circle #4 Starting Position.

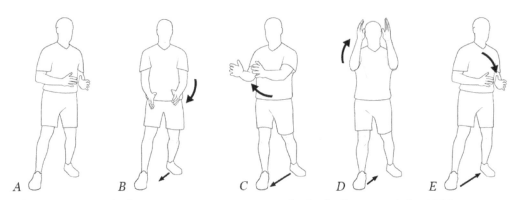

A  B  C  D  E

*Figure 19-10: Circle #3, Bottom to Top Vertical Circles + Weight Shift + Hip Turn, right leg forward.*

**Circle #4: Horizontal Circles + Kwa Squat**

1. **Starting Position**. Adjust your feet to Neutral Posture position. Sink into a Kwa Squat. Place your hands, palms down, at the Back of your Horizontal Circle. (Figure 19-11A.)

2. **Make counterclockwise Horizontal Circles, 10 repetitions**. (Figure 19-11A-E.) As you move, feel your feet and center. Before and after each Kwa Squat,

## Putting It All Together: Circles #1 through #7

balance the pressure in your feet and return your center to the vertical. After 10 repetitions, return to the Back of your Horizontal Circle.

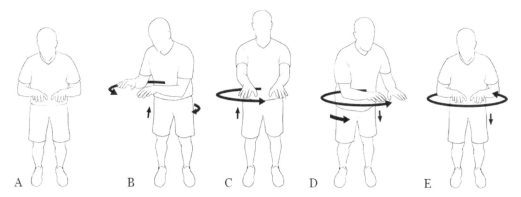

Figure 19-11: Circle #4, Counterclockwise Horizontal Circles + Kwa Squat.

3. **Change directions; make clockwise Horizontal Circles, 10 repetitions.** (Figure 19-12A-E.) As you move, feel your feet and center as described above. After 10 repetitions, return to the Back of your Horizontal Circle. Then go to Circle #5 Starting Position.

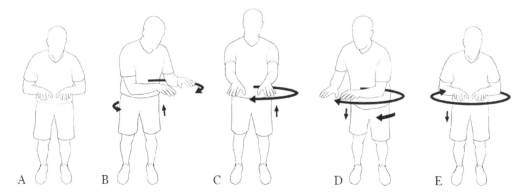

Figure 19-12: Circle #4, Clockwise Horizontal Circles + Kwa Squat.

## Circle #5: Horizontal Circles + Weight Shift + Hip Turn

1. **Starting Position, Left Leg Forward Stance.** Shift weight back. Turn your hips into your weighted leg. Place your hands at the Back of your Horizontal Circle. (Figure 19-13A.)

2. **Make counterclockwise Horizontal Circles, 5 repetitions.** (Figure 19-13A-C.) As you move, feel your feet. Feel the constantly changing pressure in each foot. Feel your center. Maintain, or correct to, a vertical posture. After 5 repetitions, return to the Back of your Horizontal Circle.

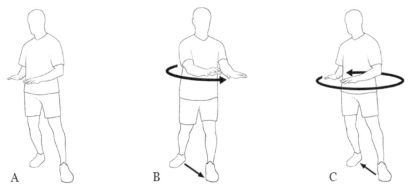

*Figure 19-13: Circle #5, Counterclockwise Horizontal Circles + Weight Shift + Hip Turn, left leg forward.*

3. **Change directions; make clockwise Horizontal Circles, 5 repetitions.** (Figure 19-14A-C.) As you move, feel your feet and center as described above. After 5 repetitions, return to the Back of your Horizontal Circle.

*Putting It All Together: Circles #1 through #7*

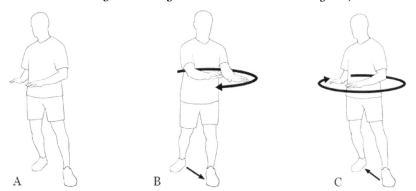

Figure 19-14: Circle #5, Clockwise Horizontal Circles + Weight Shift + Hip Turn, left leg forward.

4. **Change your stance to Right Leg Forward Stance**. Shift weight back. Turn your hips into your weighted leg. (Figure 19-15A.)

5. **Make clockwise Horizontal Circles, 5 repetitions**. (Figure 19-15A-C.) As you move, feel your feet and center as described above. After 5 repetitions, return to the Back of your Horizontal Circle.

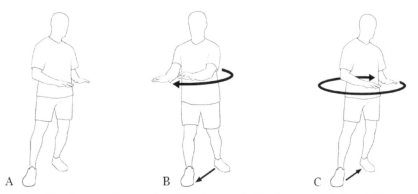

Figure 19-15: Circle #5, Clockwise Horizontal Circles + Weight Shift + Hip Turn, right leg forward.

6. **Change directions; make counterclockwise Horizontal Circles, 5 repetitions**. (Figure 19-16A-C.) As you move, feel your feet and center as described above. After 5 repetitions, return to the Back of your Horizontal Circle. Then go to Circle #6 Starting Position.

# TAI CHI FOR BALANCE

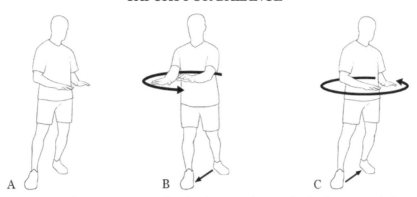

*Figure 19-16: Circle #5, Counterclockwise Horizontal Circles + Weight Shift + Hip Turn, right leg forward.*

## Circle #6: Coronal Circles + Kwa Squat

1. **Starting Position**. Adjust your feet to Neutral Posture position (feet parallel, under the hips). Sink into a Kwa Squat, hips straight ahead. Place your hands at the Bottom of your Coronal Circle. (Figure 19-17A.)

2. **Make counterclockwise Coronal Circles, 10 repetitions**. (Figure 19-17A-E.) As you move, feel your feet and center. Before and after each Kwa Squat, balance the pressure in your feet and return your center to the vertical. After 10 repetitions, return to the Bottom of your Coronal Circle.

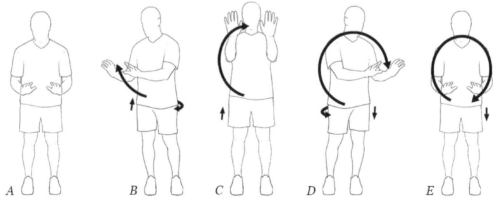

*Figure 19-17: Circle #6, Counterclockwise Coronal Circles + Kwa Squat.*

3. **Change directions, make clockwise Coronal Circles + Kwa Squat**. (Figure 19-18A-E.) As you move, feel your feet and center as described above. After

10 repetitions, return to the Bottom of your Coronal Circle. Proceed to Circle #7 Starting Position.

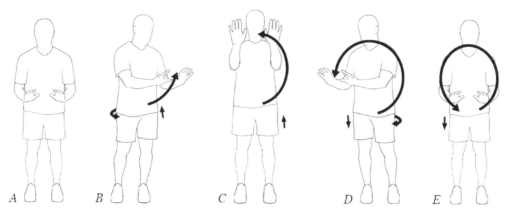

Figure 19-18: Circle #6, Clockwise Coronal Circles + Kwa Squat.

## Circle #7: Coronal Circles + Weight Shift + Hip Turn

1. **Starting Position, Left Leg Forward Stance.** Shift weight back. Turn your hips into your weighted leg. Place your hands at the bottom of your Coronal Circle (Figure 19-19A.)

2. **Make counterclockwise Coronal Circles, 5 repetitions**. (Figure 19-19A-C.) As you move, feel your feet. Feel the constantly changing pressures on each foot. Feel your center. Maintain, or correct to, a vertical posture. After 5 repetitions, return to the Bottom of your Coronal Circle.

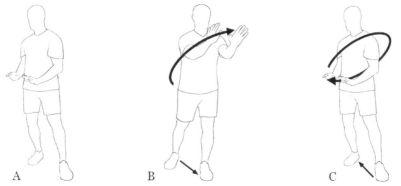

Figure 19-19: Circle #7, Counterclockwise Coronal Circles + Weight Shift + Hip Turn, left leg forward.

3. **Change directions; make clockwise Coronal Circles, 5 repetitions.** (Figure 19-20A-C.) As you move, feel your feet and center as described above. After 5 repetitions, return to the Bottom of your Coronal Circle.

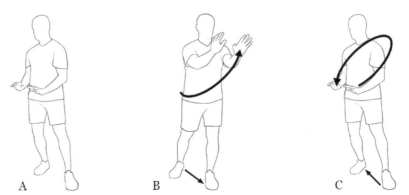

*Figure 19-20: Circle #7 Clockwise Coronal Circles + Weight Shift + Hip Turn, left leg forward.*

4. **Change your stance to Right Leg Forward Stance.** Shift weight back. Turn your hips into your weighted leg. (Figure 19-21A.)

5. **Make clockwise Coronal Circles, 5 repetitions.** (Figure 19-21A- C.) As you move, feel your feet and center as described above. After 5 repetitions, return to the Bottom of your Coronal Circle.

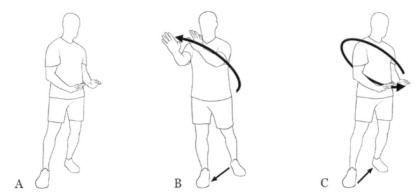

*Figure 19-21: Circle #7, Clockwise Coronal Circles + Weight Shift + Hip Turn, right leg forward.*

*Putting It All Together: Circles #1 through #7*

6. **Change directions; make counterclockwise Coronal Circles, 5 repetitions**. (Figure 19-22A-C.) As you move, feel your feet and center as described above. After 5 repetitions, return to the Bottom of your Coronal Circle.

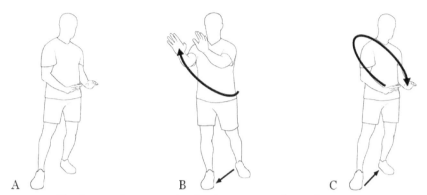

Figure 19-22: Circle #7, Counterclockwise Coronal Circles + Weight Shift + Hip Turn, right leg forward.

## Conclusion

➢ Smoothly return to Neutral Posture.

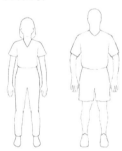

➢ **Stand in Neutral Posture for 1–2 minutes**. Notice how you feel after 140 circles, 160 Weight Shifts, 60 Kwa Squats, and 120 Hip Turns. That's a high volume of low-impact movement, all while practicing Whole Body Awareness and Precise Posture Control.

**Practice Recommendation:** Practice Exercise 32 regularly, 4–5 days per week, 1 time each day. That's just 15-20 minutes a day to feel stable, secure, and confident on your feet. And avoiding falls. Keeping you on your feet and out of the emergency room.

Remember: Follow the 70% Rule and the Don't Cause Pain Rule. If a full set feels like too much, reduce the number of repetitions per set. If 5 days per week feels like too much, reduce the number of practice days. Then gradually work your way up to a full set, 4–5 days per week.

When you're ready for a little more challenge, go to the next chapter and start Tai Chi Walking.

# Part 5

# Stepping Up the Challenge: Tai Chi Walking

In Part 5, we add **Tai Chi Walking**, the final exercises in the Tai Chi for Balance System.

A group of three exercises, Tai Chi Walking incorporates much of the material introduced in previous chapters, including all the elements of Whole Body Awareness and Precise Posture Control. On that foundation of familiar material, Tai Chi Walking ups the challenge, adding another Tai Chi movement component— **slow, deliberate steps**. Meaning, we're about to spend more time on one leg.

Spending more time on one leg, especially with slow, deliberate steps, delivers powerful benefits, including:

- Increasing the muscular work performed by the lower body, strengthening your legs and hips
- Deliberate, intentional movement and placement of the feet, refining your Whole Body Awareness
- Careful attention to maintaining an upright, relaxed, vertical posture, especially when on one leg, refining your Precise Posture Control

One other key benefit of Tai Chi Walking—You're training patterns of stepping and movement that your nervous system can reflexively activate to avoid a fall.

Part 5 includes two short chapters. Chapter 20 guides you through three Tai Chi Walking Exercises. In Chapter 21, I conclude by offering suggestions on what to do after completing Tai Chi for Balance.

# Chapter 20

# Tai Chi Walking

This chapter introduces three Tai Chi Walking Exercises:

- Single Step Forward
- Single Step Forward, Single Step Back, Single Step Forward
- Three Steps Forward and Sink

Students consistently find these exercises fascinating, fun, and challenging.

Before getting into the exercises, we'll explore a key difference between Tai Chi Walking and how we usually walk (our "normal gait"). That difference is what makes Tai Chi Walking such a terrific exercise for avoiding falls.

**Gait Analysis and Normal Gait**

Human gait analysis is a branch of biomechanics involving observation, measurement, and analysis of how people walk. There are many good reasons to study human gait, including:

- Analysis of movements and forces involved in walking
- Diagnosis of disease or other impairments affecting walking
- Evaluation of rehabilitation methods
- Evaluation of rehabilitation progress

# TAI CHI FOR BALANCE

For example, as a graduate research assistant in the University of Illinois at Chicago Biomechanics Lab, clinical gait analysis was one of the tools I used to evaluate differences in how subjects recovered from total hip replacements.[39]

In analyzing human gait, researchers typically break down a single stride (a stride = two steps) into lots of separate pieces.[40] Each piece involves different aspects of a step, including leg position, torso position, center of gravity movement, arm movements, external and internal forces. Here's a simplified breakdown of normal gait.

Our walker starts with her weight forward, with the ball and toes of her back foot still on the ground. (Figure 20-1A.) She then swings the back leg forward, moving the torso and her center of gravity forward as the leg swings. (Figure 20-1B.) She lands on the heel of the unweighted foot. (Figure 20-1C.) *Then immediately*, our walker shifts all her weight to the front leg. (Figure 20-1D.) That's a step. Our walker repeats the actions with her other leg. (Figure 20-1E-G.) All together, that's a stride.

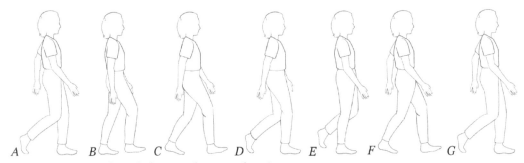

*Figure 20-1: A breakdown of normal gait.*

Our walker continues striding along until she gets where she's going.

## Normal Gait: The Problem with the Immediate Weight Shift

---

[39] Christopher C. Cinnamon et al., "Static and Dynamic Abductor Function Are Both Associated with Physical Function 1 to 5 years after Total Hip Arthroplasty," *Clinical Biomechanics (Bristol, Avon)* 67 (July 2019): 127–33, https://doi.org/10.1016/j.clinbiomech.2019.05.009.

[40] David Levine, *Whittle's Gait Analysis,* 5th edition (Edinburgh; New York: Churchill Livingstone, 2012).

I draw your attention to the immediate weight shift after swinging the leg forward and landing the heel. (Figure 20-B-D.) By immediately shifting weight, **you're committed to the step**. This happens unconsciously. We don't think about it.

At the point of the immediate weight shift you're especially vulnerable to falling. If your heel lands on ice, wet linoleum, or other slick surface, *you slip*. If a branch, rock, or other obstruction catches your foot, *you trip*. If you don't regain your equilibrium after the trip or slip, *you fall.*

To be clear, there's nothing wrong with stepping, landing a heel, and immediately shifting weight. It's functional and efficient. Humans evolved to walk like this. Once we learn how to walk, we mostly walk without giving it much thought. For much of our life, that's OK.

But, as you know from Chapter 1, as we age, falling becomes a major risk to our health. Mindlessly and immediately shifting weight after landing a heel contributes to that risk.

**Tai Chi Walking: How to Walk without Immediately Committing to a Step**

My position is this: To avoid falls as we age, we need to develop different approaches to walking. This includes incorporating exercises to strengthen our legs and hips. This also includes training to become aware of our feet and our posture. You've worked on all that since the beginning of Tai Chi for Balance.

This also includes training how to *not* commit to a step. By that I mean how to step forward, land a heel, and *not* immediately shift weight. We need to develop the awareness and skill to step forward and not commit to the step.

What happens when we combine Whole Body Awareness, Precise Posture Control, strong legs and hips, and skill in stepping forward and not committing to a step?

If we feel our heel land on a slick surface, and we avoid slipping.

If we feel an obstruction catch our foot, and we avoid tripping.

In short, **we increase our skill at avoiding falls**.

So, how do you develop the awareness and skill to step forward and not commit to the step?

Practice Tai Chi Walking!

For that, we turn to our first Tai Chi Walking Exercise, Single Step Forward, starting with the Basic Elements. First, an important Practice Note.

---

**Practice Note: Using Additional Support for Tai Chi Walking**

As you'll experience shortly, Tai Chi Walking includes slow, deliberate, controlled stepping. In doing that, you'll spend more time on one leg.

Depending on your leg and hip strength, and other factors affecting your stability, you initially may find this too difficult, uncomfortable, or otherwise beyond your 70%. Excessive wobbling, anxiety, unsteadiness are signs it's too much initially.

In that case, I recommend using extra support—what we call maintaining a "second contact point" (with the leg on the ground serving as the first contact point).

For example, you can do Tai Chi Walking next to a wall or a counter, lightly touching a wall or counter with one hand.

With practice, and as your legs and hips strengthen, you'll find you can comfortably reduce the amount of support.

---

## Tai Chi Walking #1: Single Step Forward

In this exercise, you'll train yourself to separate your step forward from the weight shift forward. It's great exercise for your legs and hips and an excellent test for your posture and alignments.

Most importantly, you're training your nervous system to respond by not shifting weight when your foot contacts an obstruction, a slippery spot, or other situation that could cause a fall.

# Basic Elements

1. **Starting Position, Left Leg Forward, weight forward.** Adjust your stance for stability and comfort. Shift weight forward. (Figure 20-2A.) Extend your hands to your sides, palms down. (Figure 20-2B.)

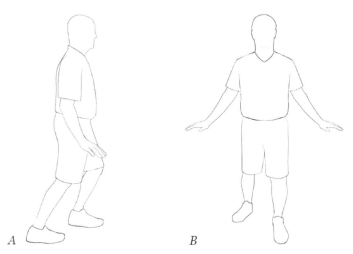

*Figure 20-2: Tai Chi Walking Starting Position.*

2. **Lift your back heel.** Keeping the ball of your back foot on the ground. (Figure 20-3A.) Pause, stabilize, and relax.

   **Note:** If you feel unstable with your heel lifted, try widening your stance. You can move your back foot out an inch or so. As we learned in Chapter 2, this increases your base of support, increasing stability.

3. **Step forward, landing the heel lightly.** Lift your unweighted foot off the ground. Smoothly move the foot forward until it's in front of your weighted foot. (Figure 20-3B.) Land the heel as softly as you can. (Figure 20-3C.) Do not shift weight. Pause, stabilize, and relax.

4. **Shift weight.** Smoothly shift weight forward. Pause, stabilize, and relax. (Figure 20-3D.) Check your alignments and posture.

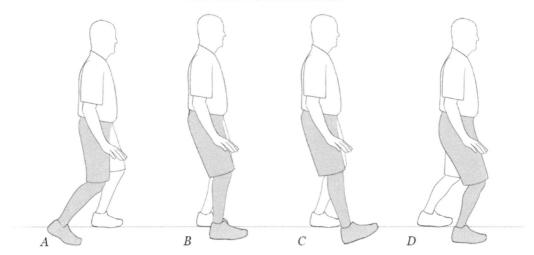

Figure 20-3: Single Step Forward, Right Leg.

5. **Repeat, starting with right leg forward.** Same instructions as above, stepping with your left leg. (Figure 20-4.)

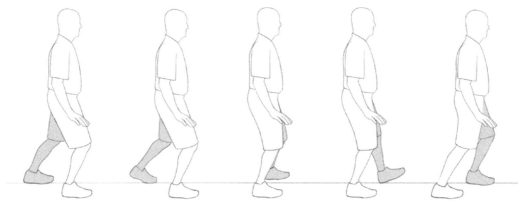

Figure 20-4: Single Step Forward, Left Leg.

As promised, in Tai Chi Walking, we separate the landing of the heel from the weight shift forward. Recognizing you've taken millions of steps and immediately shifted weight after landing your heel, this may take some practice.

As you begin that practice, I recommend you review the *Tips and Common Errors* below. Following the tips and correcting common errors will help you get the hang of the exercise in short order.

## Tips and Common Errors

*Tips*

**Maintain your alignments and vertical posture.** Recall the alignments and posture you've practiced. You aim to incorporate all of that into Tai Chi Walking. Maintaining these alignments increases your stability as you step.

**Initially, keep your steps small.** You'll find the exercise easier by keeping your steps small. For example, you could land the unweighted heel 1-2 inches ahead of the other foot. Small steps reduce the amount of time on one leg. Smaller steps also reduce the shift forward in your center of gravity, helping you feel more stable while on one leg.

Later, as you feel more stable during the exercise, you can experiment with extending your step length.

**Take it slow.** Performing Tai Chi Walking slowly delivers two key benefits. First, the slower you step, the more muscular work performed by your legs and hips. Over time, the slower you step, the stronger your legs and hips will become. Second, taking it slow gives you more time to feel what's happening as you step. This includes any tendencies to tense up, lean, or narrow your stance.

Slowing down and feeling for these tendencies helps you correct them and progress toward increased stability as you step.

**"Kiss the ground with your foot."** I love this quote attributed to the late Buddhist monk Thich Nhat Hanh: "Walk as if you are kissing the earth with your feet."[41]

I encourage you to apply that idea to Tai Chi Walking. Land your heel as softly as you can, like it's kissing the ground. This will increase the exercise for your legs and hips, and train your nervous system to separate the step from the weight shift.

---

[41] Thich Nhat Hanh and H. H. the Dalai Lama, *Peace Is Every Step: The Path of Mindfulness in Everyday Life*, ed. Arnold Kotler (New York: Random House Publishing Group, 1992).

## Common Errors

**Leg collapsing inward as you step.** When beginning to take slow steps, it's common for the unweighted leg to collapse inward during the step. (Figure 20-5A.) This narrows your stance, reducing your base of support, and making you less stable. (Figure 20-5B.) If you feel this happening, try widening your stance slightly as you step. With practice, you'll eliminate the inward collapse and maintain your stance width.

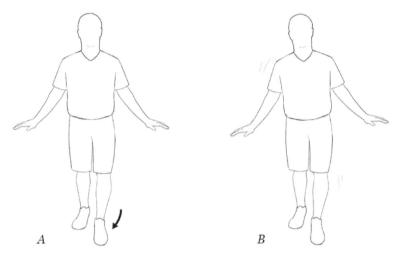

*Figure 20-5: Common Error: Unweighted leg collapsing in during the step.*

**Lifting the rear heel as you shift weight forward.** It's common initially for people to allow the rear heel to raise as they shift weight forward after a step. I encourage people to keep the back heel on the ground. In doing so, you'll get a light stretch through the Achilles tendon and calf area. If you find keeping the back heel down causes strain, shorten your steps.

With those Basic Elements, tips, and common errors in mind, let's proceed to Exercise 33.

## Exercise 33: Tai Chi Walking; Single Step Forward

1. **Getting Ready to Move.** Take a minute, or more if you like, and stand quietly before moving. First, settle into Neutral Posture. Then feel your feet, balancing the pressure in your feet. Then feel your center, aligning your center vertically.

*Tai Chi Walking*

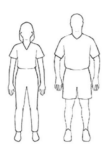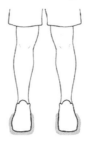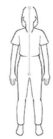

2. **Tai Chi Walking Starting Position, Left Leg Forward.** Shift weight forward. Extend your hands to your sides, palms down. Feel your feet; one loaded, one unloaded. Feel your center. Establish a vertical posture. (Figure 20-6A.)

3. **Lift your back heel.** (Figure 20-6B.) Feel for any tendency to become tense or anxious. That can happen as we anticipate being on one leg. Pause, stabilize, and relax. Feel your center. Maintain, or correct to, a vertical posture.

4. **Step forward, landing the heel lightly.** Lift your unweighted foot off the ground. Smoothly move the foot forward until it is in front of your weighted foot. (Figure 20-6C.) Land the heel as softly as you can. (Figure 20-6D.) Do not shift weight. Pause, stabilize, and relax in this position.

5. **Shift weight.** Smoothly shift weight forward. Pause, stabilize, and relax in this position. (Figure 20-6E.) Check your alignments and posture.

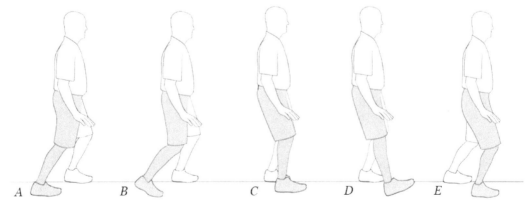

*Figure 20-6: Tai Chi Walking, Single Step Forward, right leg.*

6. **Repeat, stepping with the other leg.** Same instructions as above, stepping with the other leg. (Figure 20-7A-E.)

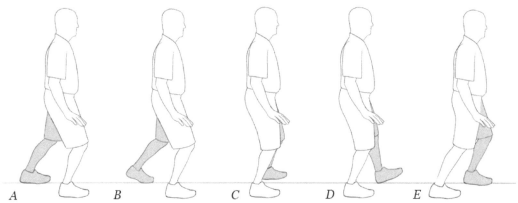

*Figure 20-7: Tai Chi Walking, Single Step Forward, left leg.*

7. **Continue for 20 Single Steps Forward.** Repeat the instructions above for a total of 20 Single Steps Forward. As needed, adjust your position in your practice space to make room for your next steps. For example, if you have space for 5 Single Steps Forward, then after five steps, turn around, and perform 5 Single Steps Forward in the opposite direction.

8. **Conclusion.** Smoothly return to Neutral Posture.

**Practice Recommendation:** Take as much time as you need to get comfortable with this exercise. You want your Single Steps Forward to feel smooth, deliberate, and controlled, all while maintaining a relaxed, stable, vertical posture throughout.

In doing so, you are continuing to develop strong legs and hips, while honing your Whole Body Awareness and Precise Posture Control. You're also training your nervous system in a new movement pattern— taking a step and ***not*** committing to that step. This becomes a key fall-avoidance technique when your feet feel an obstruction or hazardous change in walking surface.

Lots of options for incorporating Exercise 33 into your practice. For example, you could do a set of Tai Chi Circling Hands followed by Tai Chi Walking. Or you could practice your Tai Chi Circling Hands in the morning, then do Tai Chi Walking in the afternoon. I encourage you to experiment. Find what's convenient and enjoyable for you.

When you can comfortably perform 20 repetitions of Single Step Forward, try the next exercise.

## Tai Chi Walking #2: Single Step Forward, Single Step Back, Single Step Forward

In this exercise, we step up the challenge by adding a step back.

This exercise delivers all the benefits of Tai Chi Walking described above. Plus, you're training your nervous system in a new movement pattern— taking a step, not committing to that step, then withdrawing your foot. This provides a falls-avoidance technique when your feet feel an obstruction or hazardous change in your walking surface.

This technique also helps you avoid stepping in something you don't want on your shoe. In class, we call this the "Dog Park Exercise." You'll see why in a moment.

I'll briefly cover the Basic Elements, most of which are familiar from the previous exercise.

## Basic Elements: Single Step Forward, Single Step Back, Single Step Forward

1. **Starting Position, Left Leg Forward.** Adjust your stance for stability and comfort. Shift weight forward. Extend your hands to your sides, palms down. (Figure 20-8.)

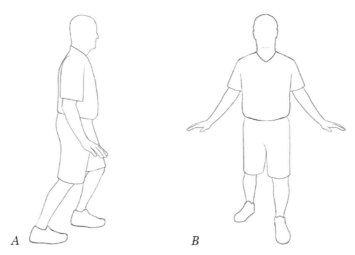

Figure 20-8: Tai Chi Walking Starting Position.

2. **Lift your back heel.** Keep the ball of the back foot on the ground. (Figure 20-9A.)

3. **Step forward, landing the heel lightly.** Lift your unweighted foot off the ground. Move the foot forward until it is in front of your weighted foot. (Figure 20-9B.) Lower the heel until it lightly contacts the floor. (Figure 20-9C.) Do not shift weight.

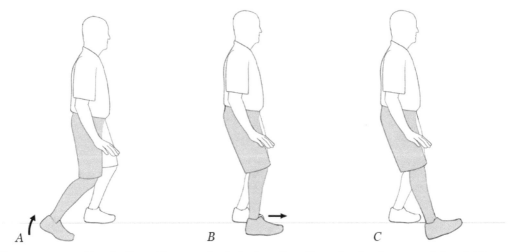

Figure 20-9: Single Step Forward, right leg, landing the heel, no weight shift.

## Tai Chi Walking

4. **Step back, landing lightly on the ball of the foot.** Lift your front foot off the ground slightly. (Figure 20-10A.) Move your foot back until it is behind your weighted foot. Lower the ball of your foot until it lightly contacts the floor. (Figure 20-10B.)

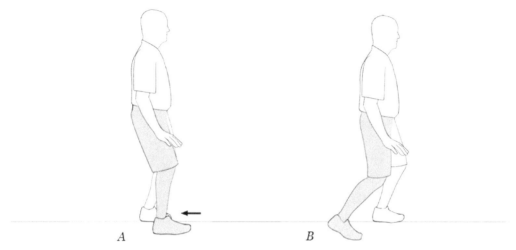

*Figure 20-10: Single Step Back, right leg, landing on the ball of the foot.*

5. **Shift weight back.** (Figure 20-11A.)

6. **Shift weight forward.** (Figure 20-11B.)

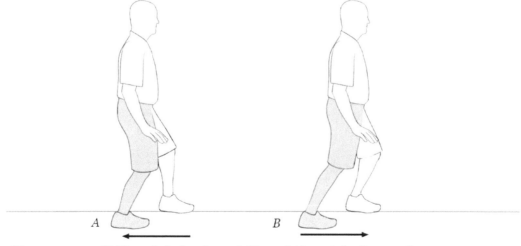

*Figure 20-11: Shift weight back, stabilize, shift weight forward.*

7. **Step forward, landing the heel lightly.** Lift your back heel. (Figure 20-12A.) Lift your back foot off the ground. Move your foot forward until it is in front of your weighted foot. (Figure 20-12B.) Lower your heel until it lightly contacts the floor. (Figure 20-12C.) Do not shift weight.

8. **Shift Weight forward.** (Figure 20-12D.) Check your alignments and posture. Pause, stabilize, and relax.

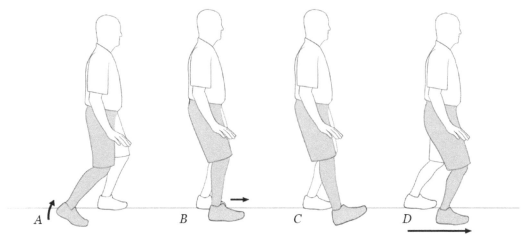

*Figure 20-12: Single Step Forward, right leg, landing the heel lightly, then shift weight forward.*

Figure 20-13 shows the movements in sequence.

*Tai Chi Walking*

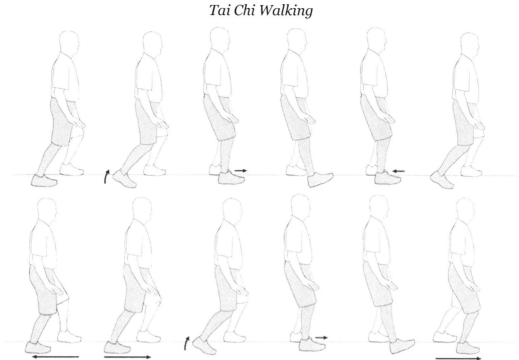

Figure 20-13: Single Step Forward, Single Step Back, Single Step Forward, right leg.

9. **Repeat, starting with right leg forward.** Same instructions as above, stepping with the other leg. (Figure 20-14.)

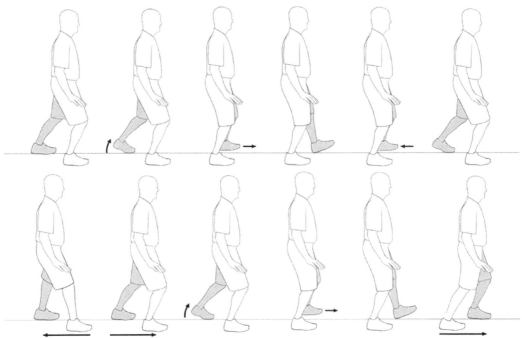

*Figure 20-14: Single Step Forward, Single Step Back, Single Step Forward, left leg.*

The tips and common errors for Single Steps Forward apply equally to this exercise. I'll add one tip you may find helpful.

## Tip

**If feel unstable stepping back, touch your toes to the ground.** Most of us find stepping back a little trickier than stepping forward—mainly because we can't see back there! If you feel unstable while stepping back, lower the toes of your unweighted foot to contact the ground. Pause, relax, and stabilize. Then raise your toes and complete the step back.

With practice, you'll find you need to lower your toes less and less. But they're there when you need them!

With that, let's proceed to Exercise 34.

# Exercise 34: Tai Chi Walking, Single Step Forward, Single Step Back, Single Step Forward

1. **Getting Ready to Move.** Take a minute, or more if you like, and stand quietly before moving. First, settle into Neutral Posture. Then feel your feet, balancing the pressure in your feet. Then feel your center, aligning your center vertically.

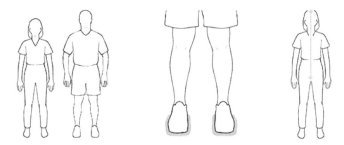

2. **Tai Chi Walking Starting Position, left leg forward.** Shift weight forward. Extend your hands to your sides, palms down. Check your alignments and posture. (Figure 20-15A.)

3. **Lift your back heel.** Keep the ball of the back foot in contact with the ground. Check your alignments and posture. Pause, stabilize, and relax. (Figure 20-15B.)

4. **Step forward, landing the heel lightly.** Lift your unweighted foot off the ground. Move your foot forward until it is in front of your weighted foot. (Figure 20-15C.) Lower your heel until it lightly contacts the floor. (Figure 20-15D.) Do not shift weight. Check your alignments and posture. Pause, stabilize, and relax.

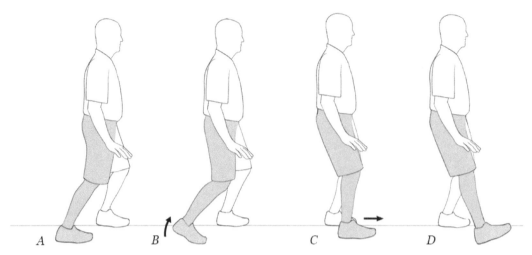

*Figure 20-15: Single Step Forward, right leg, landing the heel, no weight shift.*

5. **Step back, landing lightly on the ball of the foot.** Lift your front foot off the ground slightly. (Figure 20-16A.) Move the foot back until it is behind your weighted foot. Lower the ball of your foot can until it lightly contacts the floor. (Figure 20-16B.) Pause, stabilize, and relax in this position.

6. **Weight shifts.** Shift weight back, then forward. (Figure 20-16C-D.)

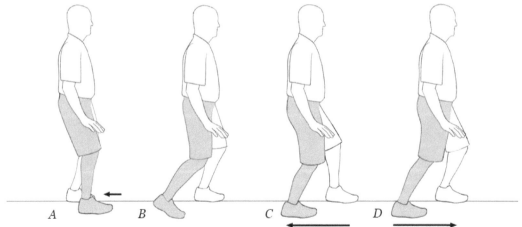

*Figure 20-16: Single Step Back, right leg, landing the ball of the foot, weight shift back, weight shift forward.*

7. **Step forward, landing the heel lightly.** Lift your back heel. (Figure 20-17A.) Lift your back foot off the ground. Smoothly move the foot forward until it is in

front of your weighted foot. (Figure 20-17B.) Lower the heel until it lightly contacts the floor. (Figure 20-17C.) Do not shift weight. Check your alignments and posture. Pause, stabilize, and relax in this position.

8. **Shift weight.** Smoothly shift weight forward. (Figure 20-17D.)

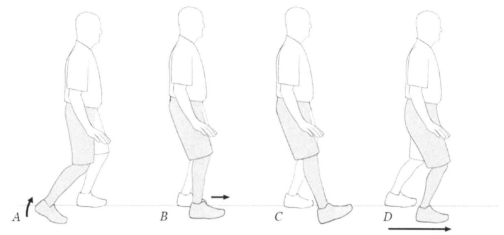

*Figure 20-17: Single Step Forward, right leg, landing the heel lightly, then shift weight forward.*

9. **Repeat with the other leg.** Same instructions as above, stepping forward, back, then forward with the left leg. (Figure 20-18.)

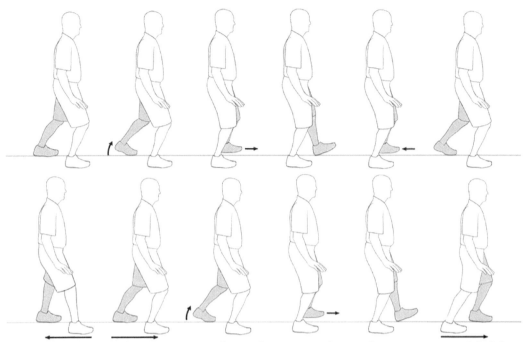

*Figure 20-18: Single Step Forward, Single Step Back, Single Step Forward, left leg.*

10. **Perform 10 repetitions.** As needed, adjust your position in your practice space to make room for your next steps.

11. **Conclusion.** Smoothly return to Neutral Posture.

**Practice Recommendation.** Take as much time as you need to get comfortable with this exercise. You want your Single Step Forward, Single Step Back, Single Step Forward to feel smooth, deliberate, and controlled, while maintaining a stable, vertical posture throughout.

When you can comfortably perform 10 repetitions of Exercise 34, try the next exercise.

# Tai Chi Walking Exercise #3: Three Steps Forward and Sink

Our third Tai Chi Walking Exercise builds upon Single Steps Forward, adding a technique for increasing stability—lowering your center of gravity.

As explained in the following Practice Note, for many of us, lowering your center of gravity in response to instability runs counter to deeply ingrained emotional and physical responses. With training, you can change those responses. Tai Chi Walking Exercise #3 provides that training.

> **Practice Note: Reprogramming Your Emotional and Physical Responses to Instability**
>
> Consider this question: How do you feel when you're unstable? When you momentarily lose your footing or wobble?
>
> Common emotional reactions include anxiety or fear. Those emotions tend to trigger physical reactions. We become tense, stiff, rising up.
>
> How does this affect our stability? Rising up, even a little, raises our center of gravity. From Chapter 2, we know that raising our center of gravity makes our structure less stable and more susceptible to a fall. The physical and emotional tension stiffens our bodies, distorting alignments and posture, impairing our ability to make small movements to recover. Our minds jump to our heads, losing track of the helpful information otherwise available from our feet and the rest of our body.
>
> In these ways, the emotional and physical responses to instability **make us more unstable**.
>
> These reactions are deeply ingrained. With training you can reprogram them.
>
> The next exercise, **Three Steps Forward and Sink**, provides that training. With practice, in response to a sense of instability, you'll relax and lower your center of gravity, increasing your stability. Another important skill to help you avoid falls.

With that, I'll briefly cover the Basic Elements of Sinking.

## Basic Elements

1. **Tai Chi Walking Starting Position, Left Leg Forward Stance.** Shift weight forward. Extend your hands to your sides, palms down. Check your alignments and posture. Pause, stabilize, and relax in this position. (Figure 20-19.)

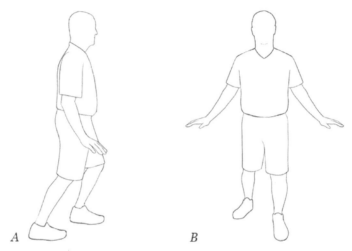

*Figure 20-19: Tai Chi Walking Starting Position.*

2. **Take Three Single Steps Forward**. (See Exercise 31 for instructions on Single Steps Forward.)

3. **After the third step, sink.** Following the third step forward, sink into your legs, by bending your legs and hips. (Figure 20-20A.) As you sink into your legs, shift approximately half of your weight back, centering yourself over your base of support. (Figure 20-20B.) Incline your torso forward as necessary to keep your weight centered. For additional stability, you can extend your arms out further. (Figure 20-20C.)

## Tai Chi Walking

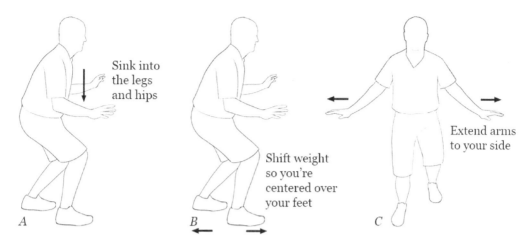

*Figure 20-20: Right leg forward, sinking after third step forward.*

4. **Stabilize.** Pause, stabilize, and relax. (Figure 20-21A.) Feel for adjustments you can make to your stance, your posture, your arms, and the depth of your sinking to feel more stable. Holding these adjustments for a moment will help pattern them into your nervous system.

5. **Recover.** When you're ready, shift weight fully forward, rising into the Tai Chi Walking Starting Position, right leg forward. (Figure 20-21B.)

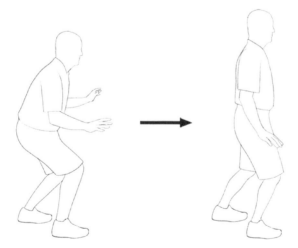

*Figure 20-21: Stabilize, then recover.*

6. **Three more Steps Forward, then sink.** Same instructions as above. After 3 steps forward, you'll end up sinking with the left leg forward. (Figure 22A-C.)

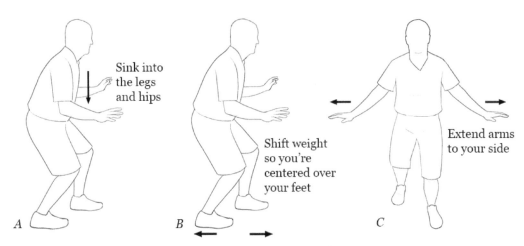

Figure 20-22: Left leg forward, sinking after third step.

7. **Stabilize.** Pause, stabilize, and relax. (Figure 20-23A.) Feel for adjustments you can make to feel more stable. Holding these adjustments for a moment will help pattern them into your nervous system.

8. **Recover.** When you're ready, shift weight fully forward, rising into the Tai Chi Walking Starting Position, left leg forward.

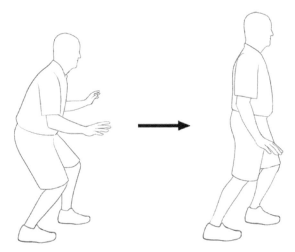

Figure 20-23: Stabilize, then recover.

Before Exercise 35, I encourage you to review the *Tips and Common Errors* below.

## Tips and Common Errors

**Tips**

**Initially, keep your sinking small.** For many people, lowering the body in the way I've just described is new. There can be a tendency to overdo it. This can cause you to lean or wobble. These actions decrease your stability.

Especially at the start, keep your sinking small. Lower the body just a little. As that action becomes smooth and balanced, you can experiment with increasing the amount of your sinking.

**Initially, take it slow.** As you sink your body, shift to even-weighted, and extend your arms, there's a lot to feel. At the start, taking it slow can help you coordinate the movements in a way that maximizes stability. You're aiming for smooth, balanced sinking.

With practice, sinking will become more familiar, eventually reflexive. As that happens, you can experiment with increasing the speed of your sinking.

**Errors**

**Leaning over.** When intending to lower the body into the legs, it's common for people to lean over, inclining the torso rather than sinking mainly by bending the legs. Leaning over tends to move the center of gravity forward, more toward the edge of the base of support, reducing stability.

To balance the pelvis moving back and down as you sink, you can incline your torso slightly forward. As with all our movements, you want to coordinate the movement of the top half of the body with the movement of the bottom half of the body.

With that, you're ready for our final Tai Chi for Balance Exercise.

# Exercise 35: Tai Chi Walking: Three Steps Forward and Sink

1. **Getting Ready to Move.** Take a minute, or more if you like, and stand quietly before moving. First, settle into Neutral Posture. Then feel your feet, balancing the pressure in your feet. Then feel your center, aligning your center vertically.

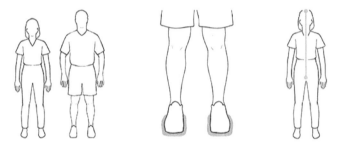

2. **Tai Chi Walking Starting Position, left leg forward.** Shift weight forward. Extend your hands to your sides, palms down. Check your alignments and posture. Pause, stabilize, and relax. (Figure 20-24.)

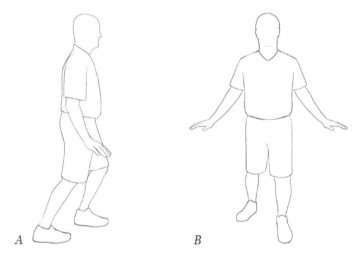

*Figure 20-24: Tai Chi Walking Starting Position.*

3. **Take Three Single Steps Forward.**

4. **After the third step, sink.** Following the third step forward, (Figure 20-25A) sink into your legs by bending your legs and hips. (Figure 20-25B.) As you sink into

your legs, shift approximately half of your weight back, centering yourself over your feet. (Figure 20-25C.) Incline your torso forward as necessary to keep your weight centered. For additional stability, extend your arms. (Figure 20-25D.)

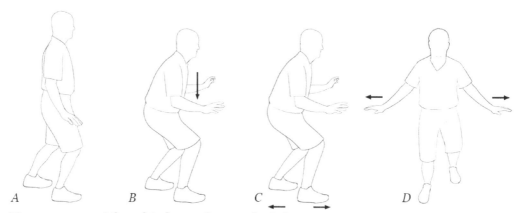

Figure 20-25: After third step forward, sink.

5. **Stabilize.** Pause, stabilize, and relax. (Figure 20-26A.)

6. **Recover.** When you're ready, shift weight fully forward, rise into the Tai Chi Walking Starting Position. (Figure 20-26B.) You're now ready to repeat the exercise with the right leg forward.

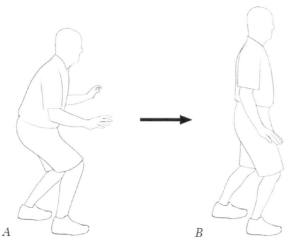

Figure 20-26: Stabilize and recover.

7. **Perform 10 repetitions.** Repeat Steps 3–6 for 10 repetitions. Adjust your direction and position in your training space as necessary.

8. **Conclusion.** Smoothly return to Neutral Posture.

**Initial Practice Recommendation.** Take as much time as you need to stabilize this exercise. You want your steps forward to feel smooth, deliberate, and controlled. When sinking, you want to feel relaxed. After sinking, you want to feel more stable.

Remember, this exercise aims to retrain our physical and emotional reactions to instability. For most, those reactions are deeply ingrained. That retraining will take some practice, repetition, and time.

You'll enjoy a major return on that investment. How? When you slip, wobble, or stumble, instead of rising up, becoming stiff, and possibly falling, you'll sink, stabilize, relax, and recover.

Then you'll continue on your way, staying on your feet and out of the emergency room.

That wraps up our journey through my Tai Chi for Balance System. You've come a long way! By now, you've accomplished the following:

- ➢ Developed greater Whole Body Awareness
- ➢ Developed increasingly Precise Posture Control
- ➢ Strengthened your legs and hips

Along the way, you've learned practical strategies for avoiding falls.

Enjoy how that feels! And keep practicing what you've learned in Tai Chi for Balance.

In the next chapter, I conclude with suggestions on where to go from here.

# Chapter Wrap-up

This chapter introduced three Tai Chi Walking exercises, building upon what you've learned in previous chapters, and upping the challenge by spending more time on one leg. Key points include:

**In Tai Chi Walking, We Separate Landing the Foot from the Weight Shift**

- In normal gait, we swing the leg forward, land the heel, and immediately shift weight forward, committing to the step. In a sense, falling onto the front leg.
- In Tai Chi Walking, when stepping forward, we smoothly, deliberately place the stepping foot forward, lightly landing on the heel. We do not immediately shift weight forward. We do not immediately commit to the step.
- In Tai Chi Walking, when stepping backward, we smoothly, deliberately place the stepping foot back, landing lightly on the ball. We do not immediately commit to the step. Then we shift weight back.

**Training Our Nervous System and Body to Move Differently**

- **Single Steps Forward** train you to separate landing the heel from the weight shift forward. So, when your stepping foot encounters a hazard that may trip you or cause a slip, you can pause and adjust to avoid the hazard.
- **Single Steps Forward, Single Steps Back, Single Steps Forward** train you to retract your foot when encountering a hazard.
- **Single Steps Forward and Sinking** train you to relax and lower your center of gravity in response to instability.

**Training Other Key Elements of Tai Chi for Balance**

- Tai Chi Walking exercises work all of the lower body, continuing to strengthen your legs and hips.
- Tai Chi Walking exercises challenge your Whole Body Awareness and Posture Control by introducing more time on one leg. While the stepping foot is airborne, our base of support is just one foot, requiring solid alignments and a vertical posture to remain stable

# Chapter 21

# Conclusion:
# Next Steps in Staying on Your Feet and Avoiding Falls

In one sense, the end of your initial training in the Tai Chi for Balance System is a beginning. For most people, completing this program involves absorbing lots of new material and feeling and moving their bodies in new ways. For the material to stabilize, to become nearly automatic, it takes an investment of time and regular practice.

To quantify that investment, you can plan on devoting 15–20 minutes per day, 4–5 days per week, for 8–12 weeks. During that period:

- Your legs and hips will continue to get stronger. You'll feel that as you walk, climb stairs, and get up from a chair.
- Your Whole Body Awareness will continue to develop. For example, as you walk around, you'll note how you're feeling your feet with increasing consistency.
- Your Precise Posture Control will continue to develop. You'll find you're increasingly aware of tendencies to lean and will reflexively move your center back to the vertical.
- Your movements will become increasingly smooth, connected, and accurate.
- You may find yourself reflexively not committing to a step when your foot contacts an obstruction or slick spot.
- You'll increasingly feel more stable, secure, and confident on your feet.

In short, your investment will return immensely valuable rewards. You will be on the path toward continuing to enjoy an active, independent lifestyle for many more years. Good for you!

A heads-up on something else you may experience.

You may find yourself really enjoying the practice of Tai Chi Circling Hands and Tai Chi Walking. After your practice, you may feel more relaxed, settled, and grounded—with a clear feeling of well-being. My students frequently report that they feel *wonderful* after their practice. If that happens to you, enjoy it!

## Online Practice Aids

A quick reminder—As a purchaser of this book, you have access to practice videos. Just press play and follow me!

In these videos, I lead you through several of the individual exercises. I also lead you through a set of Circles #1–#3, a set of Circles #1–#5, and a full set of Circles #1–#7.

In each of the videos, I provide cues to help you remember key points from the associated lessons. To access the guided practice videos, go to https://www.chicagotaichi.org/tai-chi-for-balance-guided-practice-videos/

For those who like online learning, I encourage you to check out my Online Tai Chi for Balance Course. It includes 40+ short video lessons and guided practices covering all the material in this book. To purchase immediate access to the course, go to https://www.chicagotaichi.org/tai-chi-for-balance-online-course/

## Where to Go from Here?

Here, I offer suggestions on where to go after you've completed 8–12 weeks of practice.

### Continue Practicing Tai Chi Circling Hands

For some, Tai Chi Circling Hands provides a perfect exercise program. It provides low-impact, whole-body exercise. In addition to transforming your balance and stability, regular practice of Tai Chi Circling Hands:

- ➢ Relieves chronic tension and stiffness in the shoulders, neck, and back
- ➢ Delivers the health benefits of light to moderate aerobic exercise
- ➢ Helps you release stress, relax, and become more calm and grounded

Plus, you can do it virtually anywhere. No special equipment required!

*Conclusion: Next Steps in Staying on Your Feet and Avoiding Falls*

**Explore a Tai Chi Form**

Many of my students and clients start with Tai Chi Circling Hands and then progress to the more sophisticated movements of a Tai Chi form. There are lots of options for learning Tai Chi, including classes, workshops, and online programs.

If you like my step-by-step style of instruction, check out my Online Tai Chi for Beginners Course. It includes 20+ video lessons covering all the material from a live 10-week session of the Tai Chi Level 1 classes we teach at Chicago Tai Chi. To purchase immediate access to the course, click here:

https://chicagotaichi.mykajabi.com/offers/2UDNL2DF/checkout

**Train with Me or My Colleagues**

As of the publication date, I continue to teach live classes each week, all of which are streamed online. I also provide one-on-one instruction for private clients in-person in Chicago and across the US online.

For more information on how to train with me, go to https://www.chicagotaichi.org/

**Enjoy More Physical Activity**

As the benefits of Tai Chi for Balance accrue, you will find that you can enjoy more activities, feeling stable, secure, and confident on your feet. Continue to apply your Tai Chi for Balance skills in your other activities. Follow the 70% Rule and the Don't Cause Pain Rule, and continue to feel your feet and center. Get moving and enjoy it!

**Thank You!**

In closing, thank you for purchasing this book. I am passionate about helping people realize the powerful health benefits of Tai Chi, Qigong, and meditation. I wish you the best as you take control of your health, avoid falls, and enjoy an active, independent lifestyle.

**A Quick Favor**

If you enjoyed this book, please help spread the word and leave a review on Amazon.

# About the Author

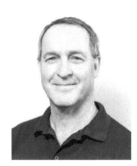 Chris Cinnamon is a lawyer, author, exercise physiologist, wellness expert, and head instructor at Chicago Tai Chi. Chris holds a law degree from the University of Michigan, a Master of Science in Kinesiology from the University of Illinois at Chicago, and is certified as an exercise physiologist by the American College of Sports Medicine. Chris lives and teaches in downtown Chicago, leads seminars and workshops throughout the US, and is passionate about sharing the powerful benefits of Tai Chi, Qigong, and meditation for the body, mind, and spirit. Chris is the author of *Tai Chi for Knee Health: The Low-Impact Exercise System for Eliminating Knee Pain* (2019) and *Tai Chi for Balance: How to Stay on Your Feet and Avoid Falls* (2023). For more on Chris's teaching and writing, go to https://www.chicagotaichi.org/.

# About the Illustrator

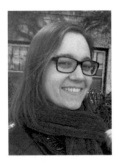Elizabeth Moss is a Chicago-based scientific illustrator. Her work ranges from anatomy illustrations to optics diagrams. She has a Bachelor of Fine Arts in Illustration from Columbia College Chicago, and a Master of Science in Biomedical Visualization from the University of Illinois at Chicago. Elizabeth is passionate about creating images that are easily understood, even when the concepts are complex. Her work has been published in scientific journals, including as cover illustrations. *Tai Chi for Balance* is her second book collaboration. For more about Elizabeth and to view her portfolio, go to https://www.emoss-illustration.com/